How to Hack Your
Vagus Nerve

*Exercises to dramatically reduce
inflammation, anxiety and
trauma with vagal stimulation*

Angelina Power

Table of Contents

Introduction

T he human body is involved. It consists of a lot of organs that work together for the proper functioning of the body. By this, any malfunction or dysfunction could lead to fatal effects. One of these is the 10th cranial nerve, otherwise known as the Vagus Nerve. The Vagus nerve is the most extended and most complex of the twelve pairs of cranial nerves that stem from the brain. It has two bunches of sensory nerve cell bodies and connects the body to the brainstem. The vagus nerve serves as a link between the abdomen to the brain, neck, heart, and lungs. The nerve is numbered, CN X.

This insightful book painstakingly gives an extensive account of the vagus nerve, which is the tenth cranial nerve. It stresses that the vagus nerve is the main component of the automatic nervous system that performs a vital role in regulating metabolic homeostasis. Also, it plays a role in the neuroendocrine-immune axis to maintain homeostasis through the afferent and the efferent pathways.

This groundbreaking book that defies the norm of orthodox medicine takes us on a journey to understand the processes involved in the fixing of the VNS device to the chest of the patient to correct disorders such as epilepsy. In order to give you a brief insight into the book, the VNS device is inserted subcutaneously in the upper chest. Afterward, electrode lead wire is attached to the left mid-cervical vagus nerve via another cut in the remaining area of the neck. The cable is then passed through a subcutaneous tunnel and linked to the pulse generator. This method has proven to be effective in treating epilepsy, and it had close to a hundred percent success rate

Most times, people that subscribe to VNS or plan to accept are in a dilemma on the workings of **VNS.** Affixing the device to the body of the patient requires an intricate process in which the doctor puts the patient to sleep. A device is then inserted into the body to arouse the vagus nerve. The doctor can get to this connection through a little incision in the neck. After the simulator has been put in, it is then encoded to produce pluses of electricity at uninterrupted intervals. However, this rests on how much the patient can take. Usually, the simulator is controlled according to specifications.

Also, there are some techniques involved in VNS. These techniques include the left cervical method of VNS and the right cervical functions of VNS.

Furthermore, there is another novel way of performing VNS, which is the Transcutaneous form of Vagus Nerve Stimulation. This method is viable because Patients can use the transcutaneous method of vagus nerve stimulation themselves. Depending on the technique used, it can be applied unilaterally or bilaterally. However, it is essential to note that there is no fixed method of how the transcutaneous form of vagus nerve stimulation can be used.

VNS is not only limited for the use of treating epilepsy, it also has some affiliation with depression. The basis for examining vagus nerve stimulation as a method of treating depression is based on several studies. For instance, in animals, it has been discovered that vagus nerve stimulation has antidepressant effects. Vagus nerve stimulation has an encouraging impact on moods in epilepsy. The vagus nerve has links to the cortical-limbic-thalamic-stratal neural link that is crucial to cognitive an emotional function linked to depression.

Also, it is crucial to note that the vagus nerve is a significant constituent of the automatic nervous system, and it plays an essential role in the control of metabolic homeostasis. Also, it plays a critical role in the neuroendocrine axis to sustain homeostasis through its efferent and afferent pathways. Arousal of receptors expressed on immune cells by pathogen-associated molecular patterns induces an upsurge of anti-inflammatory effect via its afferent pathways.

As mentioned above, a malfunction or injury to the Vagus nerve could have terrible effects. One of the impacts of the breakdown of the Vagus nerve is epilepsy. Epilepsy occurs when the brain produces electrical signals in a distorted way. Vagus Nerve stimulation is as critically explained above, is a method by which epilepsy could be treated. Although epilepsy is one of the effects of an injury or a deficiency to the vagus nerve, this book aims at using therapy (polyvagal healing) to restore normal vagal function. Many people have problems that relate to their automatic nervous system, in which most medical doctors advise them to go for surgery. However, this book aims at using therapeutic means to correct those problems, particularly by accessing the healing power of the 10th cranial nerve.

Furthermore, some exercises can be performed when trying to restore normal vagal function. Some of these exercises include the Basic Exercise, whose aim is to boost social engagement. It changes the position of the atlas, neck vertebra, and the axis. In addition, it raises the mobility of the neck and the spine as a whole. Also, it boosts the way blood flows to the brainstem, where the five cranial nerves crucial for social engagement come from. This can have a good effect on the ventral branch of the vagus nerve and the other four cranial nerves. Basic Exercise has some directions on how to use it. If strictly adhered to, it is a viable way of restoring social engagement.

Another exercise contained in this book is the Neuro-Fascial Release method. It has been grown based on the understanding on the principles of biomechanical craniosacral therapy, osteopathy, and connective-tissue release. It has been used with massive success for many years, and many therapists have learned it. This technique takes less than five minutes to perform, highly effective, and requires no physical effort. It could be used on anyone. This innovative Exercise that defies orthodox medicine can be used as a substitute for the Basic Exercise mentioned above. It is expressly valuable for treating babies, children, and adults on the autism spectrum who lack the required verbal communication skills to absorb instruction about the Basic Exercise when it might be hard to communicate with them and have them adhere to your guidelines.

Also, in touching on massage for migraines, this book informs us that Migraine headache pain has four different pattern illustrations. In some drawings, the location of trigger points on the surface of the muscles that can be massaged in order to release tension in the affected muscles is indicated. These drawings show the four typical patterns of migraine pain. Look for the model that best fits the symptoms of your migraine; this will make it easier to identify the part of the muscle, which is tight and where to massage it.

In these drawings, each pattern has trigger points that have been marked. The trigger points are areas on the surface of a muscle where there is a high concentration of nerve endings. These trigger points are sometimes thicker or harder than other muscles, and those that are often found to be released are painful when pressure is applied on them.

Again, the salamander exercise is one of those that restores social engagement of the vagus nerve. It progressively boosts the flexibility in the thoracic spine, releasing movement in the joints between the person's ribs and the sternum. This raises the person's breathing capacity, reduces forward head movement head by bringing your head back into better alignment, and reduces an abnormal spine curvature.

Most of the fibers of the vagus nerve are afferent (sensory) fibers. This means that they bring information back from the body to the brain, while only meager percent are motor fibers that carry instructions from the brain to the body — some of the afferent fibers from parts of the ninth cranial nerve. Also, the tenth cranial nerve screen the amount of oxygen and carbon dioxide in the blood. By boosting our pattern of breathing with these drills, we can tell the brain through the afferent nerves that we are safe and that our visceral organs are performing at optimum. Consequently, this brings about the ventral vagal activity.

Another exercise that can restore social engagement that will be discussed extensively in this book is the twist and turn Exercise for the trapezius. This Exercise helps in improving the tone of a flaccid trapezius as well as balancing its three parts with the other two sections. It's aids also includes improving breathing, lengthening the spine, and correcting forward head posture (FHP), which in turn alleviates back and shoulder pains. The Exercise which requires less than a minute to do it. It is not only for FHPs; it can benefit anyone.

That's not all; there is also a very effective method of restoring social engagement, which is the four-minute natural facelift. This treatment makes the facial muscles to relax, improves the functions of the cranial nerves V and VII. This method has numerous benefits some of which are; it brings about a youthful liveliness, helps to put life in the muscles of expression, makes very high cheeks a little flatter and brings out flat cheekbones, increases the circulation of blood to the skin of the face, boosts your sense of empathy by making your face responsive to interactions with others, helps you to smile often and naturally, and improves the circulation of the skin.

The person trying to do this technique must be able to see a clear reflection of themselves. In the case of doing it yourself, you have to hold a mirror to your face while if it being performed on another person, it is advised that you give the person the mirror to stick to their face so that the face can be watched and the changes can be tracked, Afterwards, take crucial notice of the skin around the cheekbone. It is advisable to do one side of the face first to be able to compare the two sides. The differences should become more apparent when you talk or smile.

You want to know more. You don't have to wait any longer as this insightful manual on accessing the therapeutic power of the 10th cranial nerve (Vagus Nerve) will take you through the disorders associated with the Vagus nerve while highlighting the various corrective exercises by which you can use to access the healing power of the Vagus Nerve. Have a good read.

Chapter 1: Vagus Nerve Stimulation

T he vagus nerve is the tenth cranial nerve, and it arises from the medulla, and it carries the afferent and efferent fibers. It is a significant component of the autonomic nervous system that plays an essential role in regulating metabolic homeostasis, and it also plays a role in the neuroendocrine-immune axis to maintain homeostasis through the afferent and the efferent pathways. It is a mixed nerve that contains 20%efferent fibers that send signals from the brain to the body and 80% afferent fibers that send messages from the body to the brain.

Vagus nerve stimulation (VNS) is generally used in describing any method that arouses the vagus nerve. Vagus nerve stimulation is a neuromodulator treatment used for the treatment of people that has medically refractory epilepsy. It is a medical treatment that has to do with delivering electrical impulses to the vagus nerve, which is produced by a programmable pulse generator. It is an adjunct treatment for some types of intractable epilepsy and major depression. VNS has to do with an epilepsy treatment where a doctor puts a pulse generator into the body to stimulate the vagus nerve, which runs from your brain to your torso. VNS treats the condition of patients with medically intractable partial epilepsy without respective surgical options or those whose surgery is contradicted for medical reasons.

The vagus nerve is associated with different functions and brain regions. From researches that have been done, the many uses of VNS include; treatment of various anxiety disorders, obesity, chronic heart failure, prevention of arrhythmias, which causes sudden cardiac death, alcohol addiction, among others. As of 2018, VNS has been discovered to be able to treat fibromyalgia and migraine.

The VNS device is a generator as small as the size of a matchbox, which is implanted under the skin below the person receiving the treatment's collarbone. Lead wires from the generator are tunneled up to the patient's neck, wrapped around the left vagus nerve at the carotid sheath, where it delivers electrical impulses to the nerve. The most frequent clinical usage of this method has to deal with the surgical procedure of putting a commercially available pulse generator. The surgery is done under anesthesia and is an outpatient method. This device is inserted subcutaneously in the upper chest. The electrode lead wire attached to the left mid-cervical vagus nerve via another cut in the left area of the neck. The cable is passed through a subcutaneous tunnel ad linked to the pulse generator. It is possible that there are surgical complications during the procedure, and it includes wound hoarseness and infection. However, the number of patients who experience this are relatively insignificant.

At this juncture, it is essential to then give a complete overview of the Vagus Nerve Stimulation process. This is because a lot of people do not know about it and are therefore scared of the resultant effects that might come from It. Sit back and learn insightfully;

How is VNS done?

It requires an intricate process in which the doctor puts the patient to sleep. Afterward, a device is inserted into the body to arouse the vagus nerve. This device is the size of a silver dollar, and it is inserted under the skin in the upper part of the chest. When this is done, a connecting wire is run under the skin from the stimulator to an electrode connected to the vagus nerve. The doctor can get to this connection via a small incision in the neck.

How it works

After the simulator has been put in, it is then encoded to produce pluses of electricity at uninterrupted intervals. However, this rests on how much the patient can take. The setting of the simulator can be controlled to specification.

It is worthy of note that VNS has some intricate techniques which require specialist attention. These methods are going to be critically discussed below:

Techniques involved in Vagus Nerve Stimulation

Generally, there are some methods of VNS. Although they are practical and relatively safe, they have their adverse effects that could result from the process. However, this seldom occurs as the process is an intricate procedure that follows the best practices. This is because the tenth cranial nerve is extremely crucial for the social engagement of the body. By this, we shall be examining those techniques and their possible side effects. Have a good read.

Left Cervical Vagus Nerve Stimulation

The small computer encodes the pulse generator stimulation parameters through a programming device put on the skin on top of the invention. On the flip side, VNS is mostly related to stimulation. By this, it is experienced for brief and intermittent periods. The adverse effects that are possible from VNS are mostly linked to the body structure drained by the vagus nerve. However, most of the fibers are afferent, and the electrical pulses are circulated from the point where the device is attached to the brain. Stimulation from the left mid-cervical vagus nerve most times causes alteration of voice, dysphagia, neck pain, cough, and dyspnea. It is believed that the left cervical VNS minimizes cardiac problems such as asystole, which is facilitated by the right vagus nerve. The parameters of stimulation can be controlled to reduce the adverse effects. However, when it comes to making stimulation tolerable, it has to do with severe cases of stimulation. It has been proven that VNS is safe, well-tolerated in pediatric patients, and is effective. There have been no specific risks that have been cited when VNS had been used during pregnancy. The procedure is safe and is well-suited with electroconvulsive treatment and psychotropic drugs. Comprehensive body scans cannot be done with Vagus Nerve Stimulation implants. However, detailed scans of the head are realizable by using a receiving coil.

Right Cervical Vagus Nerve Stimulation

Proper cervical vagus nerve stimulation decreases the activity of seizures in animals. Evidence has shown that this is also true in humans. However, it is not affirmed whether the right cervical VNS is valid for the treatment of depression. A particular vagus nerve stimulation device has been built to treat heart failure. This device is put in the wall of the chest. It is linked to the right cervical vagus using a method programmed to preferentially activate the vagal efferent fibers that are intended to affect heart function. This device perceives the rate at which the heart beats and shuts off at a fixed brink of bradycardia.

Transcutaneous forms of Vagus Nerve Stimulation

Three sensory nerves called the auriculotemporal nerve, great auricular nerve, and auricular branch of the vagus nerve supply the outer ear. The auricular branch of the vagus nerve exclusively provides the meatus and concha. A transcutaneous vagus nerve stimulation focuses on the cutaneous receptive aspect of the auricular branch of the vagus nerve. The result of applying an electrical stimulus to the left cymba conchae is an activation of the brain that is similar to that of the left cervical

Transcutaneous electrical nerve stimulators can be used for the treatment of epilepsy, and they were approved some years back. They could be used by situating contact electrodes in the part of the cymba conchae. It is possible for patients to use the transcutaneous method of vagus nerve stimulation themselves. Depending on the technique used, it can be applied unilaterally or bilaterally. However, it is essential to note that there is no fixed method of how the transcutaneous form of vagus nerve stimulation can be used.

Vagus Nerve Stimulation and Depression: Extensive Analysis

The basis for examining vagus nerve stimulation as a method of treating depression is based on several studies. For instance, in animals, it has been discovered that vagus nerve stimulation has antidepressant effects. Vagus nerve stimulation has an encouraging impact on moods in epilepsy. The vagus nerve has links to the cortical-limbic-thalamic-stratal neural link that is crucial to cognitive, and emotional function linked to depression.

Tolerability of using Vagus Nerve Stimulation

The tolerability and adequacy of vagus nerve stimulation in depression are linked to that seen in epilepsy. The side effects that were most common included alteration in voice, neck pain, and dyspnea among others. Typically, they were moderate in severity and often got better as time went on by fine-tuning the Vagus Nerve Stimulation. Vagus Nerve Stimulation was not linked to suicidal thoughts or attempted suicide. Over time, depression-related suicidal symptoms reduced as time went on.

Inflammatory biomarkers, the heart, and depression

Extensive studies have shown that depression is an independent risk factor for the growth of cardiovascular disease. This comorbid depression boosts the morbidity and mortality of patients with heart disease. In addition, depression contributes to the risk of having cardiac arrhythmias. Heart failure that results from tachycardia is convoyed by changes in autonomic tone. This results in a rapid rise in heart rate and reduced heart rate variability. Often, autonomic malfunction in heart failure is linked with neurohormonal activation.

The neuro-endocrine-immune axis and the vagus nerve

The vagus nerve is a significant constituent of the automatic nervous system, and it plays an essential role in the control of metabolic homeostasis. Also, it plays a vital role in the neuroendocrine axis to sustain homeostasis through its efferent and afferent pathways. Arousal of receptors expressed on immune cells by pathogen-associated molecular patterns induces an upsurge of anti-inflammatory effect via its afferent pathways

Chapter 2: Polyvagal Priming: Being Calm After Trauma

After trauma, calmness can be very elusive. Although many of us are told that we can get over it and that it is an experience in the past, we don't entirely return to our usual selves. This is why an experienced researcher has, for many years, carried out extensive research, to gain insight into the sympathetic and parasympathetic nervous systems that control stimulation and relaxing. These two make up the autonomous nervous system. Also, it has been discovered that the parasympathetic system is composed of two parts that create a hierarchy of three methods that respond to safety and danger.

Rest: Parasympathetic Nervous system

The parasympathetic nervous system aids digestion, repair, and rest. It reduces the heart rate and breathing rate, boosts the flow of blood to the digestive organs, and boosts the function of the immune system. In contrast to sympathetic nerves that come from the mid and lower spine, parasympathetic nerves have a direct source; this is the brain. Parasympathetic nerves are also called the tenth cranial nerve, which is our primary subject of study, as you will see later in this book.

Action: Sympathetic Nervous System

The sympathetic nervous system aids movement. It controls flight or fights reactions. Also, it controls functions that deal with exertions of the muscles. In addition, it increases the heart rate, dilates the pupils of the eyes, and boosts the heart and breathing rate. To achieve a balance, the supply of blood to the digestive decreases. Also, the function of the immune system is reduced. When the adrenals secrete hormones, the sympathetic nervous systems activated. The adrenals are located at the top of the kidney, and once the hormones are moving, it takes some minutes for them to clear from the body. This is why a rush of adrenalin does not wane immediately; we realize that there is no more danger.

It has been proven by the polyvagal theory that there are two sets of vagus nerves. These two are long nerves that run directly from the brain stem to the lungs, heart, and digestive system. They are bilateral, going down the left and right sides of the body. They have somewhat different functions because they are not entirely symmetrical. They have fibers that are sensory to the brain and those that perform motor functions from the brain. These fibers create feedback loops that control the organs and make them function optimally in their correct range

Dorsal Vagus

The dorsal vagal nerves begin at the back of the brain stem. They are unsheathed and by this, send slow and imprecise signals. A high tine signal on these nerves causes heart and breathing to slow dramatically. The body goes limp or plays dead. This is different from a tense "can't do" freeze created by conflicting impulses. The nervous system resorts to the dorsal vagal freeze when it evaluates that this is our only hope for survival or when it has given up on survival.

Chapter 3: Deep-rooted and Innovative facts about Anatomy: The Polyvagal Theory

Conquering Health Problems

A lot of people struggle with health problems. However, their problems are likened to the mythical Greek story of Hercules and Hydra. Hercules was on a mission to kill Hydra, a snake like water beast with many heads. For every head cut, two grew in its place. Her breath was also poisonous. Hercules had been given a golden sword by Athena, a powerful god who accompanied heroes to battle. Luckily for Hercules, one of Hydra's heads was mortal, and he was able to kill her. This story is typical of how many of us treat the symptom of one health problem only to have another crop up. The society relies on biomedical drugs and surgery, which are powerful and effective. A process like surgery leaves scars that could hinder the movement of muscles on adjacent areas. Because the autonomous nervous system regulates vital functions of the body, abnormal functioning of the cranial nerve and the vagus nerve could lead to a lot of consequences.

Common Problems Related to Cranial-Nerve Dysfunction

Chronic physical tensions

- Lump in the throat

- Cold hands and feet
- Tenseness after stress
- Arthritis
- The strain of eyeballs

Emotional issues

- Low energy levels
- Crying easily
- Frustration
- Excessive fantasizing
- Sleeping problems

Heart and lung problems

- Hyperventilation
- Hypertension

Visceral-organ dysfunction

- Digestion problems
- Gluttony
- Diarrhea

Immune-system problems

- Flu
- Allergies

Behavioral Problems

- Asperger's syndrome
- Increase in drinking or smoking

Interpersonal Relationships

- Disinterest in sex
- Trust issues

Mental Issues

- Excessive worrying
- Difficulty remembering

Other Problems

- Skin Problems

Lots of people have one or two of these symptoms frequently. These problems can be classified as physical, mental, emotional, and behavioral. In this context, we are citing differences by grouping the symptoms. It distracts one from the observation that the underlying physiological cause is the same.

Comorbidity is the scientific name for when a person experiences these symptoms at the same time. If the symptoms occur frequently, it is advisable to treat it, but if it seldom happens, it is not a problem. Instead of using separate pills for different symptoms, maybe we can find one treatment method that can eliminate all the signs. All the issues in the list above apart from dorsal vagal activity can be resolved by making the ventral vagal nerve and other nerves necessary for social engagement to function correctly. The cranial nerves and the role they play is often overlooked in modern-day medicine. Lots of people are not aware of what the brainstem is and where the nerves originate, among other things. However, the truth is that if we can get five nerves that support social engagement to function appropriately, we stand a good chance of getting rid of most of the symptoms listed above.

Chapter 4: An Insight into the Autonomous Nervous System

T he essential bodily function of the nervous system is to ensure survival. It comprises the brain, brainstem, enteric nerves, cranial nerves, and spinal nerves. The autonomous nervous system is made up of the elements of the brainstem, parts of some spinal nerve, and a bit of the cranial nerve.

Cranial Nerves

There is a difference between cranial nerves and spinal nerves. The brainstem is connected to the nose, eyes, ears, and tongue by some cranial nerves. The brainstem comes from the brain. It lies under it and is the beginning of the spinal cord. Each of the twelve cranial nerves has pathways on both sides (left and right).

The vagus nerve was given its name because it is long and passes through the body from the brainstem to the chest and abdomen to control visceral organs. It passes through the pharynx and larynx, lungs, heart, organs of digestion, and kidneys. Also, it was named from the Latin word "Vagus," which means vagrant wanderer. It helps to control a lot of functions that are necessary for Homeostasis in the body. Several of the cranial nerves support non-stress states compared to the sympathetic chain, which supports stress states and survival. Apart from ensuring rest, the cranial nerves also enable the senses of sight, smell, taste, hearing, and touch on the face.

Roman numerals number every cranial nerve. They are numbered according to their location, and they extend from a semi-circle on each side of the brain. The vagus nerve is numbered, CN X.

Functions of the Cranial Nerves

Cranial nerves have various features, and the first look at them would make their tasks seem related. In Anatomy, this is not usually noted as the twelve cranial nerves have a common attribute; they are all involved in helping us chew, swallow, and eliminate undigested food as waste. Cranial nerves control and monitor the following things;

- secretion of enzymes and acids in the mouth and stomach
- production of bile, storage of bile
- production of digestive enzymes
- regulation of the movement of undigested food from the stomach to the colon
- The release of gall and pancreatic enzymes into the duodenum

It is crucial to start the discussion of cranial nerves by noting the role they play in the digestive process. Afterward, we will examine other functions of the cranial nerves, such as control of the kidney and bladder, heart and respiration, and sex and reproduction.

If you have primary or little knowledge about cranial nerves, you don't need to rack your brain to recall the function of each. What is important is getting a general view of the features these nerves regulate and the state of social engagement. However, if you know about it, this will broaden your knowledge.

The olfactory nerve numbered CN I was the first cranial nerve to develop, and it enables our sense of smell. The smell is vital for humans as it helps in finding food and determining whether it is edible.

The way we respond to smell is compelling and based on instincts. Smells have various emotional effects on us; for instance, a baby has to feel its mother. The origin of the nerve fibers of the olfactory nerve in the nose has a direct pathway to the forebrain.

The olfactory nerve is the only cranial nerve that transmits signals from the sensory organs to the brain without an intermediary synapse. This part of our "old brain" is crucial for forming memories and survival. This explains why the strongest memories deal with the smell. CN I, the optic nerve, comes from the brain and helps or vision, thereby helping us find food.

Moving our eyeballs in different directions makes us see more. Three cranial nerves control the small muscles that move the eyeballs, and they allow us to roll our eyes in different directions. Also, we can see more if we use the neck muscles to move our head. The spinal accessory nerve controls the muscles that help us run our head to look in different directions. This allows us to search for food and distinguish if a portion of food smells sweet or not. Although these processes are reasonable, it is crucial to taste food properly. This involves mixing the food with saliva, which is controlled by trigeminal and glossopharyngeal. Saliva increases our ability to taste things and starts the process of digestion. To mix saliva with food, we use the trigeminal nerve to innervate the muscles for mastication, opening and closing the jaw, and grinding the grain; the hypoglossal nerve to move our tongue to shift the food in the mouth, and the facial nerve to relax and tighten the muscles of the cheek to facilitate emptying the food back to the grinding surfaces of the teeth.

To taste food, the taste buds on the tongue are used to connect the three branches of cranial nerves; the facial nerve, glossopharyngeal nerve, and the vagus nerve. By this, if the food does not taste good, we can quickly spit it out. When swallowing, the tongue flips chewed food mixed with saliva to the esophagus. The esophagus is a muscular tube that transports food from the throat to the stomach, contracting rhythmically just like intestines. The upper third of the esophagus is innervated by the ventral branch of the vagus nerve, while the other parts of it are innervated by the dorsal vagus branch.

The cranial nerves help in the search for food in diverse ways. A lot of animals locate prey using their finetuned organs of hearing. The auditory nerve is considered to be the only cranial nerve that aids hearing. However, in mammals, the trigeminal and facial nerves play essential roles in listening and understanding human speeches by controlling the middle-ear muscles

Cranial Nerves and function

- **CN I:** Olfactory Nerve- Smell
- **CN II**: Optic Nerve- For sight
- **CN III**: Oculomotor Nerve- Controls some eyeball muscles
- **CN IV:** Trochlear Nerve- Controls some eyeball muscles
- **CN V:** Trigeminal Nerve- for chewing, swallowing and hearing
- **CN VI:** Abducens Nerve- Control some eyeball muscles
- **CN VII**: Facial Nerve secretions- for chewing and hearing
- **CN VIII**: Acoustic Nerve- For the hearing
- **CN IX**: Glossopharyngeal Nerve- Swallowing
- **CN X**: Vagus Nerve (old and new)
    1. Old: Controls organs such as the liver and gall bladder. It is also responsible for the movement of food through the intestine.
    2. New: Innervates and controls the upper third part of the esophagus and most of the pharyngeal muscles
    - **CN XI**: Spinal accessory nerve- responsible for the turning of the head and broader vision field
    - **CN XII**: Hypoglossal Nerve- Movement of the tongue.

Apart from other functions of the cranial nerves, the visceral afferent of cranial nerves gathers the information that pertains to safety, threat, health, pain, dysfunction, illness, and danger from our physical organs.

Social Engagement and Cranial Nerve Dysfunction

Typical human behavior is considered to be an expression of positive social values. By this, our actions should be beneficial to us and others. When we are socially engaged, we make more sense, and people understand us better. A lot of us are socially engaged most times, but sometimes, go into the state of fight or flight or withdrawal. If our autonomous nervous system is strong enough, we will bounce back. For those who are not socially engaged, they lack resilience to bounce back instantly from a state of social engagement, thereby becoming stuck in dorsal vagal states. In this state, it is hard for people to understand the motivation, behavior, and values; often, actions seem irrational and counter our best interests. It could have destructive effects and make life difficult for the sufferer and those around them.

Cranial Nerves necessary for social engagement and problems that might arise when they don't function properly

Trigeminal Nerve and Facial Nerve secretions
The fifth cranial nerve has various motor and sensory functions. These include controlling the muscles of mastication and receiving impulses from the sensory nerves in the face. Dysfunction of the trigeminal nerve can make someone's face deadpan. The fifth and seventh cranial nerves have interrelated functions. The seventh cranial nerve innervates the face while trigeminal is a

sensory nerve to the skin of the face. We are shown a feel of the face when facial expression changes. Both nerves play significant roles in listening and understanding, which is crucial for social engagement.

 The seventh cranial nerve innervates the smallest nerve in the body (Stapedius). It shields the inner ear from noise. By reducing the volume of sounds in a mother, the stapedius allows the baby to hear the mother's voice. Being easily disturbed by background noises could be a signal that your stapedius is not functioning correctly. Other signs of a dysfunction of the stapedius are hyperacusis and tensor tympani innervated by the trigeminal nerve. When the tensor tympani tighten, tension is increased, thereby diminishing sound. This helps in the reduction of noise when we eat.

Orthopedic braces and tooth extractions could cause a dysfunction of the fifth and seventh cranial nerve, particularly in adults. A slight misalignment of the facial bones between the sphenoid and palatine bones can pressurize both nerves.

The sphenoid bone is centrally situated in the skull. Temples are made up of the outer surfaces of the bone. A person hit on the temples while boxing will knock out. The bone has a saddle-like depression where the pituitary gland rests. A dislocation between and palatine bones could result in dysfunction of the nerves of the face and middle-ear. When this occurs, the entire social nervous system is blocked. The fifth cranial nerve goes to the face while the seventh goes to the muscles of the face. To correct the dysfunction of these, some methods kindle the fifth and seventh cranial nerve. Although, when you practice the techniques, you will notice an improvement; it is crucial to consistently practice those techniques, especially if you've lost your natural smile.

Medial and lateral pterygoids are innervated by Trigeminal, arise on the sphenoid bone, and help to open and close the jaw. A displacement of this could cause overbite, underbite, or overbite.

Glossopharyngeal Nerve, Vagus Nerve, and Spinal accessory nerve

One of the two branches of the vagus nerve comes from a structure called the nucleus ambiguus in the brainstem, together with the glossopharyngeal nerve and spinal accessory nerve. The dorsal branch of the tenth cranial nerve comes from the floor of the fourth ventricle close to the back of the brainstem. The two branches of the vagus nerve and the ninth, eleventh nerve, and jugular vein pass through the jugular foramen. Fibers of the ninth and eleventh cranial nerve weave themselves into the tissues of the vagus nerve. When there is a symptom indicating dysfunction of one of these nerves, the other two are most times affected. Therefore, an improvement in vagal function will lead to an increase in others.

Treatment of Cranial nerves

The method of treating cranial nerves is different from spinal nerves. Therapists use chiropractic-like methods to treat spinal nerves. However, to restore the function of cranial nerves, a different approach is needed. It is called cranial osteopathy. This process requires a detailed and extensive knowledge experience to understand the work and the methods accurately. The biomedical approach was developed by Alain Gehin, and he has taught his approach to many students around the world.

Stretching of the soft-tissue within the skull and spine is another method of treating cranial nerves. The dura mater is a tube of connective tissue that extends from the skull to the tailbone. Also, it contains the brain, cerebrospinal fluid, and the spinal cord.

Biodynamic craniosacral therapy is the third method of treating cranial nerves. It aims at maximizing how the cerebrospinal fluid that circulates the brain and spinal cord moves and brings nourishment to the tissues, helping them to get rid of metabolic waste. Biomedical methods hasten release by using the flow of the cerebrospinal fluid contained in the Dural membranes of the skull and spine. The therapist holds the head of the patient with a very light touch while being focused on the little movements of the cranial bone.

Nerves of the spine

Lots of people suffer from a herniated that presses on the spinal cord. Dysfunction of the spinal nerve could also cause paralysis. Chiropractic or osteopathic treatment could be used to ease compression of the spinal nerve. In contrast with osteopaths that use a gentle approach, chiropracts use high-velocity techniques to change the position of a vertebra. Other treatment methods include yoga, calisthenics, and physical therapy, among others. If these techniques do not work, you may feel inclined to use surgery. Unfortunately, surgery never gives relief as there is growing research that the relief surgeries provide is in the short-term.

A vital function of the spinal nerves is that they facilitate the movement of our body by contracting and relaxing various muscles. Also, messages to the spinal nerves stem from the brain and go through the spinal cord.

More than one branch of spinal nerves goes to any muscle. By this, should there be any malfunction, the muscles are still going to be able to function, though not optimally by using the signals from other nerves.

Sensory and motor fiber nerves give a feedback loop that allows us to tense a muscle while the sensory fibers send information to the brain about changing tension levels in the muscles at the same time. This will enable us to regulate the tensing of muscles. If the body is in a state of stress, all the muscles are tense as compared to when it is at rest.

Spinal Sympathetic link

Branches of the spinal nerves go to specific structures in the body like the skin, muscles, viscerotomes, ligaments, fascia, and fasciatomes. Instead of a single nerve innervating one muscle, there is an overlap to enable other tissues to innervate the same muscle. The nerves from the thoracic vertebrae T1 and T4 go to the heart, T5 and T8 go to the lungs, T9 to the stomach, and T10 to the kidneys. Most of the sympathetic link which goes to the head and visceral organs are followed by arteries to their endpoint.

Enteric Nervous System

This is a network of nerves that connects the visceral organs. These nerves are interwoven with the physical organs and the connective tissues. It has been herculean for anatomists to trace their pathways and functions. The only guess is that they aid visceral organs to communicate with one another to make digestion easy.

Chapter 5: The Polyvagal Theory: Three Routes of the Autonomous Nervous System

T ypically, the functions attributed to the autonomous nervous system were the control of various several visceral "automatic" functions. Traditionally, the model of relaxation was based on the sympathetic and parasympathetic circuits. In contrast to the sympathetic nervous system that was seen as a response to threat or fear, the parasympathetic nervous system was modeled for relaxation.

The Polyvagal Theory begins by knowing that the vagus nerve has two distinct vagal nerves that come from two different places. We get a precise representation of the way the autonomous nervous system works if we view the three neural circuits of the autonomous nervous system; the ventral branch of the vagus nerve, spinal sympathetic chain, and the dorsal branch of the vagus nerve. They control our body functions to maintain Homeostasis.

The activity of the spinal sympathetic chain helps us to fight or avoid a threat. This owes to the tense muscles that allow us to move quickly. Also, higher blood pressure is required to pump blood into the tight muscles. Low blood pressure is enough to pump blood into soft tissues. However, when extreme, low blood pressure can cause people to faint. A handshake gives an insight into the state of a person's autonomous nervous system. When a person has a very tight handshake, it is caused by a chronic activity in the sympathetic spinal chain. For a person with a limp handshake, it is characterized by overactivity in the dorsal vagal unit. However, if the handshake is right, the ventral branch of the vagus nerve is predominant.

The Autonomous Nervous system and Homeostasis

The neural circuits that control the nerves can be likened to a thermostat linked to a heater and an air conditioner. When the thermostat sees that it is too cold, it turns on the heater, vice-versa. In the same vein, mammals need to maintain body temperature by upper and lower limits, and the sensory nerves provide information about body temperature to the neural circuits.

The three parts of the autonomous nervous system work hand in hand to regulate the organs and help us to adapt to the environmental and balance conditions of the body. The polyvagal theory can also be used for problems like digestion and reproduction, which we might consider beyond our control.

The three neural pathways of the Autonomous Nervous system (ANS)

The social engagement nervous system is the first part of the ANS. It deals with activity in the ventral branch of the vagus nerve and four other cranial nerves. This activity has a calming and soothing effect. The ventral branch of the vagus nerve promotes love, satisfaction, and joy.

The spinal sympathetic chain is the second of the ANS's neural pathways. It activates when our survival is threatened. At this time, we can make extra effort to respond to the threat. The spinal sympathetic chain deals with emotions of fear or anger, which can manifest in behaviors such as fighting or feeling to overcome the danger.

The dorsal branch of the vagus nerve is the third pathway. This is activated when we face a crushing force. At this point, we immobilize, making us helpless and hopeless, among other things. In this state, we also withdraw and shutdown.

The two-hybrid circuits

In addition to the three pathways of the ANS, there are two fused states made up of various combinations of two or three neural circuits. This state is a fusion that supports mobilization without fear, which we need when we engage in competitive sports. In sport, it combines the effects of two neural circuits; the spinal sympathetic chain and the social engagement circuit so that we can play safely within rules and avoid hurting each other.

Hybrid of two neural circuits

In this state, activity in the dorsal branch of the vagus nerve, when combined with that of the ventral branch of the vagus nerve, supports intimacy. This is the state we can call mobilization without fear.

The Vagus Nerve

Emotional and physical well-being are closely related. If you have a headache, it is difficult to be happy. On the other hand, if you have had a good meal, slept well, and exercised, among other things, we feel revitalized and robust. However, lots of people do not know that the proper functioning of the vagus nerve is essential for feeling emotionally stable, healthy, and revitalized, among other things.

Historical recognition of the Vagus Nerve

The anatomy of the nerves deals with the location of the nerves in the body in relation to the muscles, bones, skin, and visceral organs, while the physiology deals with the function of those nerves. For the past century, these two disciplines have found their way into the education of almost all health care professionals in the western world. The vagus nerve was first recorded by a Greek physician, Claudius Galen (130-200AD). Over the years, medical doctors and healthcare professionals have built on his observations, and they have concluded that the autonomous nervous system consists of two divisions; the sympathetic and parasympathetic, which innervate the nervous system.

Polyvagal Theory

Porges gave a different model of the autonomous system. Although his concept was similar to the older model, he focused on three divisions of the Autonomous nervous system, which will be discussed below.

Two Branches of the of the Vagus Nerve.

The dorsal and vagal branches of the vagus nerve come from different places in the brain and the brainstem, have different pathways and have different functions. They are separate and distinct as there is no relationship between them. There was no distinction between the two branches of the vagus nerve before the polyvagal theory. The ventral nerve was lumped under the heading of the tenth cranial nerve. By this, there has been a long-term confusion in trying to understand the autonomous nervous system. The polyvagal theory informs us of the difference between the two branches of the vagus nerve. The ventral and dorsal nerves come from different locations. The ventral nerve comes from the ventral side of the brainstem while the dorsal nerve arises in the floor of the fourth ventricle.

The two branches of the vagus nerve can bring about immobilization. This is in contrast to the sympathetic nerve that brings about flight or fight. However, the states of immobilization are associated with types of behavior.

Effects of activity in the ventral vagus circuit

Mammals, including humans, have attained a higher, complex nervous system that includes dorsal and vagal channels. Note that it is only mammals that have the ventral circuit. To activate the circuits, the individual must be and feel comfortable in whatever environment they are. When active, the ventral circuits give rise to social engagement. Social engagement is more intricate than just relaxing. When in the ventral state, we relax, we are not in fear of anything, and we are stress-free, making us free to be immobile. On the other hand, when we are not engaged socially, we can either experience fright or flight or be frozen and depressed.

It is important to note that activation of the sympathetic nerve is not limited to when we are frightened or want to run. When we are safe, and our nervous system is functioning normally, the sympathetic nerve is activated slightly on every in-breath, causing the blood pressure to rise and the heart to beat a little faster. At this point, our pulse feels a little stronger. However, when we breathe out again, the heart rate and pressure decrease, and the pulse feels softer.

Therapists can train themselves to use their fingertips to feel this regular slight change between the mild activation of the spinal sympathetic chain and the ventral vagal unit. If there is no change, it means that there is nervous system dysfunction.

Flight or fight

This response affects our physiology when it comes to survival in the face of a threat. At this time, the muscles are tense, and the heart rate rises to pump more blood to the muscles. Also, our bronchioles dilate, thereby increasing the amount of oxygen in our lungs, blood, and cells. Waste products associated with cell metabolism are eliminated when we breathe better. Reptiles, for instance, engaging its stress state, can move with immense speed and power. This same spinal sympathetic nervous system allows humans and other humans to use the stress state as a defensive strategy by fighting or running away from fear. For instance, playing video games could put your nervous system in a state of fight temporarily, and addiction to it could put our bodies in that state permanently.

New Ways of Understanding Stress

Although a lot of people talk about being stressed, a lot of them are actually in a state of dorsal vagal activity; they are depressed. This could be caused by a traumatic incident in the past. The Polyvagal Theory describes their state as activation of the dorsal branch of the vagal nerve. Accordingly, they could begin to suffer from lethargy.

The three circuits of the autonomous nervous system have a step-like progression from one state to the next. The ventral vagus branch is at the top of the ladder, followed by the spinal sympathetic chain and the dorsal vagal circuit, which is at the bottom of the ladder. At the two lower levels, the ventral branch of the vagus nerve inhibits. Vagal circuit activity moves a person directly from shutdown and emotional depression to the ventral vagal state. Next comes the spinal sympathetic circuit. Activity in this circuit inhibits the dorsal vagal circuit. Running, swimming, or other forms of exercise that stimulates fight or flight exertions often help to bring out of depression. A lot of antidepressant drugs work in that way. By chemically stressing the body, they temporarily activate the spinal sympathetic chain. However, antidepressant medications do not bring us to social engagement, and they can have undesired effects.

Chapter 6: Neuroception and Faulty Neuroception

N euroception was thought up by Stephen Porges. He coined it to describe how neural circuits differentiate if a situation is safe, threatening, or dangerous. It is a process through which our autonomous nervous system assesses processed data from our senses about our environment and body.

The process of Neuroception takes place in the nascent parts of the brain beyond our awareness. It can be equated to a watchdog that is always on guard, which allows us to focus on things other than survival, sound sleep, and rousing us when intrusions could hinder our survival. By these signals from neuroception from neural circuits that are well defined are activated to support social engagement and friendly behaviors when we are safe.

A lot of people experience neuroception when they get to the sixth sense and know that they are threatened or are in danger without consciously knowing how they knew.

Survival and Faulty Neuroception

Neuroception makes us able to contact information that we do not pick up with the conscious part of our minds. When it functions optimally, it is the right gift and can aid our survival. In contrast to conscious perceptions, it works faster. On the flip side, neuroception could be defective. When it is defective, we could find ourselves in trouble. At this point, we distort what is going on as we do not have a clear perception. Faulty neuroception is caused when the neural circuit from perception to behavior is defective. For instance, the reaction of a person to a safe situation might be that of a threatening situation. When this occurs, then there is faulty neuroception.

The causes of faulty neuroception vary. First, our perception may be blinded by lethargy, fear, jealousy, and anger. It is possible also to be locked in traumatic memory. Again, it could be caused by shock, low blood sugar, hunger, pain, and illness. For instance, you could be feeling healthy and be triggered suddenly by something that makes you recall a traumatic experience in your past and react to this as if it were it were happening presently. In actual sense, we might not be experiencing that threatening situation, but our nervous system may be stuck in the past. Also, faulty neuroception could be caused by positive experiences like falling in love.

Typically, the nervous system should be flexible. This enables our defense mechanism to adapt to the present situation and support different kinds of situations. In the case of chemical interference, processed data comes in from the environment via the senses. However, in this case, the neural circuits do not process information normally, and our physiology does not respond appropriately. Prescription drugs, as well as banned and recreational drugs, put us in an unusual physiological and experimental state.

An instance of faulty neuroception caused by biomedical interference is aptly shown in the following story;

Three young ladies went for a hike on the amount that was an active volcano. The climb was strenuous, and they prepared well for the hike. In their backpacks, they had a map, pocketknife, first aid kit, and compass. Also, they had helmets to protect them from falling rocks, goggles in the event of an ashfall, sunscreen, functional boots, lightweight sweater, and sunglasses because of the intense sun. They began the climb very early, and the weather forecast had predicted a mild, sunny, and bright day. Soon enough, because of the sun and their exertions, they became warm, and they had to splash water on their heads.

The temperature of the body is controlled by neural reaction mechanisms that work primarily by the hypothalamus, the part of the brain that processes processed data from necessary body sensors. When overheating begins in the body, several physiological changes occur. When the temperature is over 37°C, the nerves to the blood vessels close to the skin make the blood vessels expand. This causes vasodilation, and it makes more blood to get to the small capillaries in the skin. Close to a third of the blood vessels in the body can circulate in the skin and is cooled by the surrounding air at the skin surface. Also, sweat cools the body as its moisture evaporates.

As they climbed, the weather suddenly changed; clouds formed and it began to snow. Immediately, they put on their sweaters to avoid the cold. Unfortunately, this wasn't enough, and they hadn't brought rain gear along. Within minutes, they were soaked.

When the body temperature drops, the hypothalamus works to conserve heat; automatic conservation of heat responses begins as well as mechanisms that generate additional heat. Epinephrine secretion is a normal response to cold. By this, the muscles tighten, thereby causing shivering. Body heat is produced from the rapid contractions of trembling muscles.

When responding to stress, nerves also cause tightening of the muscular walls of the blood by a process called vasoconstriction. This reduces heat loss by reducing the level of blood that flows from the center of the body to the hands and feet.

One of the young climbers who had chronic stress had taken his medication to suppress it. One of the effects of this medicine is to reduce blood levels of stress hormones. By this, his body could not react to the cold weather normally; he didn't shiver, blood vessels didn't shrink, arteries and capillaries remained opened, and the flow of blood to his skin was not reduced to prevent further heat loss. He could not adapt to the environment, and cardiac arrest occurred because of extreme hypothermia. The young climber died because his body could not adapt to the change in climatic conditions.

More causes of Faulty Neuroception

The survival value of a shutdown state was touched upon earlier. For instance, when the lion clenches its jaws on prey, the prey's autonomous nervous system shuts down automatically because it faces death and cannot fight back. In some cases, though rare, the lion could lose interest, thereby saving the antelope's life. As humans, we may not be threatened physically, but we are often susceptible, mentally, or emotionally. It could involve getting something done on time, solving an economic problem, resolving difficult issues in our relationships, and caring for a family member suffering from a terminal disease. We cannot just sit back and watch things happen; we have to act.

Again, it is essential to note that unlike animals, humans do not shake off their ordeals as soon as the threat is gone. Although it is normal for us to rest our nervous system and have a fresh start, most times, the effects of ordeals stick with us long after the traumatic event. The memories from this can stay with us for years and sometimes for the rest of our lives. Without overcoming it, it is possible to experience recurrent symptoms of shutdown and stress.

Irregular reactions to some stimuli can occur because one had an ordeal that involved them. The psychological trigger that causes a shutdown can be specific. The memory of this event is like an unexploded land mine waiting to explode. The reaction is activated because something reminds us of whatever caused our ordeals in the past.

Antaeus Story

The battle between Antaeus and Heracles was an exciting subject in Renaissance culture. The story goes thus;

Poseidon, the god of the sea, and Demeter, goddess of the earth, were the parents of Antaeus. It was believed that he lived on the edge of the desert. Typically, Antaeus would challenge passersby to a wrestling contest, beat them, and use their skulls in a temple Antaeus was building for Poseidon. However, the story changed when he fought Heracles. The secret of Antaeus' power was that anytime he was knocked down to earth, his mother being the goddess of the earth, would fortify him, and he'd bounce back stronger.

On realizing this, Heracles grabbed Antaeus by the waist, held him aloft in the air, and grabbed him into a bear hug. On Antaeus, side, the story had been used to teach what happens to those that do not keep themselves grounded while on the part of Heracles; it shows how one can bounce back again to win after being upset.

Sensing our Bodies

The skin and muscles of the face are innervated by the Trigeminal nerve and the Facial Nerve secretions. Stroking the face calms, us most times and eases us out of stress. Most times, people do this to themselves unconsciously. For instance, as a therapist, if you are giving your patients a massage, you could ask them to put their attention on where your hands are touching their bodies. This is very important for those who are experiencing withdrawal and dissociation. At that moment, when you have your hands on them, you are not trying to bring about any changes in their musculoskeletal structure; you're not relaxing a muscle, freeing movement in a joint, adjusting the spine, or releasing the connective tissue. Instead, your hands remain in the same place.

It is enough for you to place your hands on the patient's body, lightly touching the skin. Afterward, you tell the patient to come to grips with their awareness. When you start this, it could take some time for the patient to rid their minds of emotional and psychological clutter, bringing their attention back to their body. It is therefore advised that you repeat the process over and over again as it is a simple way of letting the patients use their senses to be grounded in their body.

Chapter 7: Trying the Ventral Branch of the Vagus Nerve: Appraisal from Observation

C onferring with Stephen Porges, social engagement involves the ability to look and pay attention. For instance, when conversing with someone, you can decipher if they are socially engaged with you or not. The facial muscles are ordered around the opening of the nostrils, mouth, and eyes. When these muscles are flat and round tighten, the skin around the opening closes. To allow more light into the eyes, more smells into the nose, and more air into the mouth, the flat, rectangular muscles attached to the round muscles pull them open. When we react emotionally, our facial expression changes as we open and close these openings.

The flat round muscle that surrounds the eye is called orbicularis oculi. Orbicularis is termed to be a muscle around a facial opening while oculi means related to the eyes. When the muscle tightens, we close the opening around the eye, reducing the amount of light in the same way the shutter of an old camera cuts down the amount of light coming through the lens to the film.

When squinting because of bright light, we tighten this muscle. Also, we stretch this muscle when we want to reduce our visual input, when there is something we don't want to see or when we want to withdraw from external sensory stimuli and ponder on our thoughts. When this muscle tightens, we move away from current visual stimuli. We may recall events from the past, picture the future, or begin to meditate.

 The tenseness of the flat, rectangular-shaped muscles above and below the orbicularis causes the orbicularis oculi to be pulled more open, thereby allowing more light to come in. An event like an eye-opener can make these muscles become tense. It enhances our memory intake and makes us conversant with things around us.

Though strange, when our eyes open, we can hear better. This is because there is a neurological link between the nerves involved in sight and hearing. For instance, when at a lecture, you tend to open your eyes more to her better. Try this; when you look at someone, look for impulsive facial expressions in the middle of their face. The presence or absence of these movements will determine whether if the flexibility of the person's emotional responses is present or not.

Facial expressions are divided into two; those that occur when we unconsciously make a face and those, we put on to show someone how we feel. Depending on how long they last, we can divide the former one into three types.

 The first one is the pattern of chronic tension, which is permanent, carved into our faces with deep wrinkles that indicate our emotional state.

The second one is less permanent and shows our current mood. As long as the feeling lasts, the pattern of facial tension remains. At this time, a person can get an inkling about how we are feeling.

In the third one, the facial muscles located between the mouth and eyes change tension up to several times per second. These spontaneous micro-changes are evident in babies or children. It is rare to see this in adults as we are mostly grounded in our moods. It is difficult for us to say that facial expression indicates a specific emotion because they occur rapidly. However, the fact that these spontaneous movements are there makes us aware that the person is open and without fear.

These quick changes can be experienced when two people, who feel safe with each other, make eye contact and allow their feelings to flow without stifling them. This is a reflection of a state of openness when our facial emotions change as rapidly as our thoughts. It is entirely different from the smile we put on when posing for a photo where we almost frown in a forced attempt to show positive feelings. For instance, look at the flow of emotions on someone's face. You'll notice that when happy, satisfied, angry, irritated, afraid, anxious, sad, or depressed, the movements of the face are slight, rapid, and mercurial. You could also consider this; does that person's emotional expression remain stuck? When they speak in monotones, are their voices flat? Or do they have prosodic changes in their voice when they speak? Most times, we tend to view people as unchanging personalities.

However, their interactions with other people are affected by their mood, which affected by the autonomous nervous system at that time. When people are stressed, they might look at us in a threatening way and may see, aggressive. Also, they might not listen, exhibit combativeness, and, most times; we might need to correct them. Those who are in a fear state avoid eye contact, make eye contact for a split second then look away. Also, their breathing might be shallow, and they might hold their breath after an in-breath. For those in a depressed state, they will tip their heads forwards or hang their heads with an expressionless face. Typically, they are slow in movement, have no enthusiasm, and do not want to engage in any conversation. Sometimes, before they do anything, they will sigh, indicating depression.

Additional tests of vagal function

As a therapist, apart from observing aspects such as these, it is best to start your treatment by testing for the ventral vagus branch. If the client exhibits ventral vagal dysfunction, you can use the methods and exercises described in part two of this book. After the client does the basic exercise, or after treating he/she with your hands, it is advised that you test again for the ventral vagal function to be sure that you have achieved the desired results.

In addition to the procedure that involves looking at the back of the throat and having the client say "ah-ah-ah," you could use another test that is effective for young children that are autistic or others in extenuating.

The second test is premised on the annotations by Mayer, Tarube, and Hering in the late nineteenth century. They observed that when the ventral vagus nerve is optimally functional, the pulse and blood pressure should be stronger and faster when breathing in than when breathing out. As a therapist, when you gain experience in treating many people, you will observe that the difference is more after they have done the basic exercise than it was before that time. People who have a more significant difference between the pulses when they breathe in and out are usually stronger and healthier, both physically and psychologically. However, it is essential to note that these tests have limitations as they are only observation-based. There are other ways of checking for a proper vagal function which are listed below

Heart Rate Variability: An objective method of evaluating Vagal function

There is increasing awareness of heart rate variability in scientific research on the autonomous nervous system. This is profound as it might help us find another way to evaluate vagal nerve function.

When socially engaged and functioning at its best, our nervous system has differences in the length of time between consecutive heartbeats. This results in a natural rise and fall of the heart rate in response to emotions, breathing, hormones, and blood pressure.

To indicate general health, Heart Rate Variability can be of much help as it represents one of the most hopeful evaluative gears to gauge autonomic nervous system activity. A proper function of the vagus nerve makes the person's heart rate variability high. Research has been growing in leaps and bounds to establish the link between high heart rate variability, health, and long life. On the flip side, when there is low heart rate variability, the autonomous nervous system goes into a state of dorsal vagal activity. When this happens, the difference in time intervals between heartbeats is non-existent, and this is a sign of low heart rate variability.

Developing scientific studies have shown a link between low heart rate variability and several psychological or psychiatric problems. For instance, heart rate variability is linked to the sensitive state. It has been found to reduce when subjected to emotional strain, post-traumatic pressure, severe anxiety, and acute time pressure. People who have issues related to worrying every day tend to have low heart rate variability.

Furthermore, low heart rate variability is connected to the loss of concentration and motor inhibition. The symptoms are mostly found in children with ADHD. Also, there is a relationship between low heart rate variability and post-traumatic stress disorder. In the physical health arena, low heart rate variability has also been theorized to be a sign of bad health in general. Here are some adverse health conditions that could be caused by low heart rate variability;

- The poor survival rate in premature babies
- Obesity
- Susceptibility to infant death syndrome
- The activity of the dorsal branch of the vagus nerve
- Diabetic neuropathy

Generally, those suffering from obesity have low heart rate variability. Although the narrative might be that obese people overeat, seldom exercise, do not want to change their behavior, among other things, some overweight people go on a diet and almost starve themselves with little or no result. For others, they work with a psychologist or hypnotherapist to improve their image.

Lots of people with sexual dysfunction visit their doctors for help or consult with a psychiatrist. A current study that concentrated on women shows us insight into women with sexual dysfunction. It shows that this condition may be connected to low heart rate variability. Some studies conclude erectile dysfunction in men. It notes that a general imbalance of the autonomous system is one of the causes of erectile dysfunction.

Heart rate variability studies have shown that low heart rate variability could cause heart damage. It has been linked with a high risk of coronary heart disease. Low heart rate variability appears to cause mortality after a heart attack. Low heart rate variability is related to an early death. This is caused by various causes, such as COPD.

COPD was the third-highest cause of death after heart disease in the USA in 2014. Abnormal breathing patterns show reduced physical and psychological health. Also, there is a link between diaphragmatic breathing and higher levels of heart rate variability. It has been discovered that those with a diagnosis of COPD have a little movement in their respiratory diaphragm, and their tests don't show ventral vagal activity.

A simple test of the pharyngeal vagus branch

The ventral vagus has many branches. This is a test for one of the branches called the pharyngeal branch, which innervates the part of the throat behind the nasal cavity and the mouth above the esophagus and the larynx. Nerve fibers from the pharyngeal branch of the vagus to the soft palate and to the pharynx. It is involved in making vocal sounds and swallowing.

The first extant writer to describe the pharyngeal nerve of the vagus nerve was Claudius Galen. He was a Greek physician, and he noted that the pharyngeal nerve provided motor nerve function for the muscle that produces the voice. He discovered this by treating a gladiator who had been wounded and had lost his voice. He found that the pharyngeal nerve had been severed on one part of his neck. He then tested his observation on pigs whose anatomy is similar to humans. He found that when cut, the pharyngeal nerve of the pigs would stop their squealing. After trying many options, it has been resolved that focusing on the pharyngeal branch is the better option.

This test gauges the movement of the levator veli Platini muscle. The condition of this branch is a good indicator of the function of other branches of the ventral vagus nerve, as well.

When the function of the pharyngeal branch is improved, it improves the role of the respiratory diaphragm. When there is a dysfunction of the levator veli Platini muscle, there is always irregular breathing. After the patient does the Basic exercise and the pharyngeal branch begins to function normally, the breath needs to be observed to be sure it has become improved, more profound and slower.

Guidelines on how to test for pharyngeal ventral branch function

These are the steps to take when performing the test for pharyngeal ventral branch function;

- Ask the person to sit in a chair
- Stand in front of the person and ask them to open their mouth so you can see the back of the person's throat
- You will see the small bulb-shaped structure that hangs down of the throat and the soft tissue arches on either side of it.
- This can be seen sometimes with light while at times, you could use a flashlight
- If the person is blocking your view of the uvula, as the person to place one of their fingers on the back of their tongue and push it down to the floor of their mouth
- Afterward, the uvula will be visible to you
- Ask the person to say ah-ah-ah-ah while you observe the arches on either side of the uvula (Normally, the sound produced should be distinct short bursts of sounds in quick succession and not a long drawn out aaaaaaaaahhhh which does not create the desired effect
- If the pharyngeal branch of the ventral nerve is functioning optimally, "ah-ah" lifts the arch of the soft palate equally on both sides.
- When there is dysfunction of the pharyngeal branch of the ventral vagus nerve on one side, the nerve impulses do not innervate the levator veli palatini muscle on that side, and the arch and the arch in the

soft palate on that side does not lift when the person says "ah."

This test can move one out of the state of stress or shut down into a ventral vagal state. After someone does these exercises or receives hands-on treatments, one should be able to observe improvement before the next test; the uvula and soft palate should now move equally on both sides.

Another test that could be used to test for the function of the ventral vagus nerve branch is the Trap squeeze test. Although it has its implications, it works perfectly with children or persons on the autistic spectrum that might have difficulty following directives.

Chapter 8: The Polyvagal Theory:
A New Archetypal for Health Care?

In general, the western approach to medical treatment is surgical and biomedical. For instance, when we complain to a doctor, and he examines us, he makes a diagnosis, writes a prescription, and sometimes recommends surgery.

Although these processes are commendable, modern-day doctors might be overlooking something. For instance, the dysfunction of the autonomous nervous system might be a cause of COPD, migraine, autism, and other health issues. Instead of focusing solely on diagnosis, there is a growing consciousness of comorbidity, which is the presence of more than one disorder that occurs together with a primary disease. The new condition could come in different ways.

The autonomous nervous system controls and supervises the proper functioning of the visceral organs and is a significant contributor in determining how good or bad our moods are going to be. Sadly, doctors do not usually test its function as they do not consider it a contributing factor; neither are they trained to know that it is a contributing factor to is crucial for our physical, emotional, and psychological well-being. It has been discovered that helping the ventral branch to function optimally often gets rid or reduces the harshness of many health issues. In truth, a malfunction of those nerves is a significant cause of life-changing behavioral and psychological patterns. Let's go into the journey of discovery to learn more about this.

Psychological and physical conditions: A Polyvagal approach

Lots of people spend a copious amount of time focusing on the adverse effects of stress without having a general idea of problems resulting from chronic activation of the dorsal branch of the vagal nerve. This is characterized by low blood pressure, fainting, difficulty in breathing, the rapid loss of energy. In cases of COPD and chronic fibromyalgia, this comes from constriction of the airways.

Building on Stephen Porge's success

A craniosacral therapy protocol was developed in 2002 by choosing a lot of Alain Gehin's methods. A proper application of these methods establishes adequate functioning of the ventral branch of the vagus nerve and the other four cranial nerves crucial for social engagement. Five hundred therapists in Denmark and Norway have been taught this protocol, and it has been successful in controlling the patients' autonomous nervous systems. In lots of cases, success has been incredible, and there have been no adverse effects.

It is important to note that there are severe challenges in teaching these progressive methods, especially to people that have no prior knowledge of the craniosacral system. Instead of following these sophisticated techniques, the best way is to follow the polyvagal theory and then give a description of how to do these methods. However, it is essential to note that these exercises should not replace medical care. However, it is hoped that it will make you healthier.

The Healing Power of the Polyvagal Theory

A lot of health problems are caused by a malfunction of the vagus nerve. However, it is essential that, as a therapist, before starting these tests, you have to first test the patient's autonomous nervous system. Afterward, you can then demonstrate and each self-help exercises. You can then check again to make sure that the changes have been achieved. If necessary, you can suggest that your client continues to do self-help in the future.

Hiatal Hernia and Relieving COPD

Lots of people have heard of chronic obtrusive pulmonary disease only recently. In fact, in our world today, it is one of the world's most common non-contractible health issues. Chronic obtrusive pulmonary disease is a health issue whose symptoms range from chronic poor airflow, coughing, and shortness of breath. Those who have this issue cannot do physical exercise and have breathing issues. Currently, COPD has the following causes; they include exposure to environmental toxins, smoking, among other things. When this happens, the reaction to this is that the body creates a surplus of fibers that wedge the airways in the lungs and bronchioles.

Often, people with this disorder find it complicated to keep their jobs which enable them to make a living. By this, they usually have difficulty planning . In addition, they could also have trouble keeping the level of their activity outside work. Therefore, they have a reduced quality of life.

Although steroids and inhalers can improve breathing temporarily, the health issue can return as soon as the steroids and inhalers wear off. Also, inhalers and steroids most times have side effects if used for a long time. This is why it is recommended for a short time. Furthermore, many people around the world living with this disorder cannot afford inhalers and steroids; by this, they cannot access them. Though sad, the truth is that there is no cure for this disorder that worsens until they succumb to an early death.

Typically, COPD becomes worse until when respiration is so limited that the patient cannot support and sustain life. Around the world, this disorder affects nearly 5% of the population, although the exact figures may be higher due to inadequate diagnosis. Some years earlier, COPD placed third on the rankings of the top causes of death after heart disease and cancer, killing more than three million people. Although trillions of dollars have been spent to get the cure, none has been reached. This leads one to ask, are we looking in the wrong places? Are there solutions that might not necessarily involve drugs or surgery?

Although some might disagree, extensive research has proven that the root cause of COPD comes from a malfunction of the autonomous nervous system. Also, it has shown that it is a health issue that can be solved by the understandings taken from the polyvagal theory.

Even though doctors and indeed hospitals do a lot of testing, they tend to ignore gauging the function of the autonomous nervous system. This is sad as patients can be checked swiftly without paying much for the ventral vagal function, which affects other body functions.

In the treatment of COPD, reinstating the function of the vagus nerve is a crucial element. By restoring the role of the vagus nerve, patients can be helped to improve their breathing in spite of the belief that this is generally impossible.

A case study of COPD and hiatal hernia

Vital capacity is a test for lung function. It is measured against the average age of other people of one's age group, regulated by body weight. Of a fact, it is possible for a person to have more than 100% vital capacity. From many years of experience, therapists have discovered that when there is a dysfunction in a visceral organ, in this case, the lungs, it might be caused by a malfunction of the autonomous nervous system serving that organ. The sympathetic nervous system, the ventral, and the dorsal divisions of the vagus nerve innervate the lungs. The dorsal vagal also gives a path to the subdiaphragmatic vagus nerve that spreads to the visceral organ beneath the diaphragm. The bronchioles are constricted by the dorsal branch of the vagus nerve, causing a reduction in the flow of air. The bronchioles are dilated by the sympathetic nervous system allowing air to flow in properly. When the ventral branch of the vagus nerve is functioning optimally, the bronchioles relax, allowing air to flow in and out of the lungs adequately.

When functioning correctly, the respiratory system tightens when you breathe in, pushing downward and laterally expanding the two lower ribs.

As a therapist, in testing for the proper functioning of the vagus nerve, it is essential to involve the patient to evaluate where there is movement in their chest or belly. In doing this, you can tell your client to lie down on their back and teach them how to do the basic exercise. By performing on the patient's body, you will surely notice an improvement in their breathing as they would be respiring without strain. Also, you will see that the patient's ribs would be expanding on the side as they breathe in. When this happens, it represents a landmark improvement for your patient who has had difficulty in breathing. Afterward, you have to check again in order to ensure that the ventral branch of the vagus nerve is functioning correctly.

Lots of researchers and medical doctors, most times, use a spirometer to test the capacity of the lungs. This often makes patients tense up when they are being tested, making them control their breathing. However, the preferable way is to evaluate functionally. For example, in a patient that has difficulty climbing up a flight of stairs, it is an indication that of how the person's breathing is impaired when he/ she has to exert themselves in performing everyday functions. When you adopt the functional process of evaluation for testing the capacity of the lungs, you will notice that the patient will be more relaxed. Also, he/she will become to breathe more deeply and slowly.

After this, the next goal for a therapist should be to improve how the patient's respiratory diaphragm moves. When this is done, you will notice that the lateral movement of the patient's ribs on the right side will increase. However, if, after doing this, you see that there is no physical lateral movement of the ribs on the left side, you can compare the right side to the left. By this, you will definitely notice that something on the left side is interfering with the movement of the diaphragm. If this is the case, it could be a hiatal hernia.

What is a Hiatal Hernia?

The stomach is situated on the left side of the abdomen. Typically, this is beneath the respiratory diaphragm. The elastic muscular tube that links the back of the mouth to the top of the stomach goes through the hiatus in the respiratory diaphragm. The ventral branch of the vagus nerve innervates the upper third of the esophagus. This allows its muscle fibers to change the length and lift or lower the stomach. However, it must be noted that the medical view of hernia does not consider the role of the vagus nerve.

When the vagus nerve is functioning optimally, the esophagus lengthens and relaxes, causing the stomach to move down a little bit into the abdomen as the diaphragm tightens when we breathe in. Typically, as the diaphragm comes down and goes up freely along the esophagus, the contents of the chest remain above the diaphragm, and the contents of the abdomen remain below the diaphragm. However, when there is a vagal malfunction, the upper third of the esophagus tightens and shortens, pulling the stomach up against the underside of the respiratory diaphragm.

In severe cases, the esophagus can be so tight and short that it pulls the stomach against the diaphragm. By this, it forces the opening of the diaphragm and pulls part of the stomach into the chest. This is called hiatal hernia.

Acid reflux is also an additional symptom, apart from the difficulty in breathing, that marks those that have hiatal hernia. Acid reflux or heartburn occurs when the stomach comes up against and burns the back of the throat. Other signs of hiatal hernia include eating small meals instead of three regular meals, feeling bloated, among other things.

Normal breathing involves the upward and downward movement of the diaphragm. However, with some breathing problems such as cold lungs and asthma, it has been discovered that the shortened esophagus is a significant factor that hinders normal breathing. In fact, it is the primary cause of many breathing issues. When the stomach is pulled in to it, the diaphragm cannot come down freely when breathing in.

Treating a Hiatal hernia

There is an osteopathic method of treating hiatal hernia, and it works efficiently as a self-help exercise. The first step is to teach the patient how to do the Basic exercise. Afterward, the simple osteopathic method can be used to pull down the patient's stomach, lengthen, and relax the esophagus. By employing this method, lots of health issues like shortness of breath, pulmonary fibrosis, and asthma can be eradicated.

The stomach is on the left side of the abdomen, beneath the rib cage. The first step is to place the tips of your fingers on one hand lightly where the stomach is. The belly is soft and palpable, and you should be able to feel it if you extend the tips of your fingers slowly and gently into the muscles of the abdomen. You only need to contact the top of the surface of the stomach, and under no circumstances should it be painful. Once the patient experiences pain, you should stop immediately. Pull it down gently towards the feet until you can see a sign of resistance. Usually, this happens after pulling it about one-half-inch. Hold it at the point of little resistance until the esophagus relaxes. It is not necessary to exert any force, although you might be tempted to do so. Once your fingers are on top of the stomach, you will signal the nerves for the esophagus to lengthen, and the stomach will come down in the abdomen. Thus, it will make room for the respiratory diaphragm to come down when breathing in.

Usually, a sigh or swallow goes with this moment of relaxation. When this happens, it feels as though the muscular resistance to the stomach dissipates. Instantly, the person will be able to breathe easily.

As a therapist, it is recommended that in addition to treating hiatal hernia, you address other tensions in the patient's visceral organs that could hinder breathing. In addition to doing the Basic technique, the patient should also do visceral-massage techniques. He/ she could also do some movement exercises. If strictly adhered to, within a space of twelve weeks, the patients should be able to ride a bike. As time goes on, the patient will be able to do more exertions than he/ she would have done before doing those exercises.

Most attempts to treat COPD have been using the wrong approach as they have failed to take cognizance of the fact that the problem can be linked to a malfunction of the vagus nerve. The bronchioles are constricted by the dorsal branch. This makes it difficult for air to get into the lungs. The constriction is essential for the immobilized state of shutdown. For example, a crocodile that had just had a big meal must lie still to allow the meal digest. However, if not properly monitored, it could become a problem for people who want to function well in their everyday life. Using the Basic Exercise to trigger the function of the ventral branch takes people out of the dorsal-vagal state of shutdown. By this, their bronchioles are no longer constricted.

Combined with the stretching of the esophagus, the Basic exercise takes a few minutes. Its effect is instant, as there is no prescription medicine required. Also, it does not have adverse effects.

Diaphragmatic Breathing

A significant part of social engagement is good diaphragmatic breathing. Normal breathing involves the upward and downward movement of the diaphragm. In order to know what is happening in patients that have disturbed breathing because of the activity of the dorsal branch of the vagus nerve, place your hands lightly on the sides of the chest at the level of the last two ribs. When there is diaphragmatic breathing, you will detect a lateral movement of the lower two ribs on both sides. However, in the case of hiatal hernia, you will feel the lateral movement on the right side but nothing on the left.

In case of not being able to breathe in with a standard lowering of the respiratory diaphragm, you have to find alternative ways to create space for the expanding lungs. A common way to do this is to lift the upper ribs and shoulders. This is called high costal breathing. Breathing patterns like these are linked with fear, panic, and anxiety.

Inhaling using the muscles of the abdomen is another typical pattern in non-diaphragmatic breathing. At times, when we are short of breath, the belly is distended, soft, and flabby. The muscles of the abdomen are very soft, and when they go slack, the intestines come down, pulling the lungs down. This is sometimes interpreted as a good sign and called belly breathing because the breath can be seen going down into the abdomen. However, it does not deal with the tightening of the respiratory diaphragm. Those who breathe this way hold their muscles of their stomachs when they breathe in. At this point, their abdominal muscles feel hard. This manner of breathing is linked to anger.

Typically, the abdomen and chest enlarge and contract in a rhythmic manner. The lower two ribs move to the sides, down, and back with expansion. The five upper ribs swing out to the sides. This lateral movement is equated to that of the handle of a bucket. The next group of ribs above those lift upward, together with the sternum in action described as the pump handle

A loss of optimal tonus in the diaphragm also leads to the loss of proper tonus in our musculoskeletal system. At this point, we tend to collapse into our bodies. Also, we exhibit the breathing pattern of someone who is showing depressive behavior. On the other hand, if we tighten the diaphragm and push it down onto our gut, we exhibit the breathing pattern of one who is angry.

The vagus nerve has sensory and motor fibers that affect and are affected by the movements of respiration. There are four times as many sensory nerve fibers in the respiratory branch of the vagus nerve. This is because there are motor efferent nerves that are continually monitoring the function of the respiratory diaphragm. In order to facilitate relaxed and efficient breathing, the proper role of the motor fibers of the ventral vagus nerve is crucial. When there is a malfunction of the respiratory diaphragm and does not come down when we breathe in, we make use of muscles triggered by either our spinal sympathetic sensory link or our dorsal vagal circuit. What this means is that a breathing pattern that fails to make proper use of the diaphragm will communicate through the sensory nerve fibers that we are facing a threat or are in danger. This is an instance of how feedback from sensory branches of cranial nerves impacts the state of our autonomous nervous system.

CN XI, Trapezium, and SCM: Shoulder, Neck, and Head Pain

Apart from being one of the five social engagement nerves, the spinal accessory nerve performs a unique muscular function. It innervates the sternocleidomastoid and trapezius. These two are large muscles in the neck shoulder. They are the only skeletal muscles below the head and face that are not innervated by spinal nerves. If either of them is severely flaccid or tense, it will respond in a different way to massage treatment and movement training than any other muscle in the body

Shoulder problems happen to be one of the most common forms of musculoskeletal problems. A malfunction of the eleventh cranial nerve could lead to pain and stiffness in the shoulders and neck. Sometimes, by improving the function of the tenth and eleventh cranial nerve with the Basic Exercise, one can get rid of pain in the neck and shoulders. After performing the exercise to get rid of stiffness in the neck, we might want to try other methods to treat different problems that a malfunction of these muscles can cause. The Basic exercise had the ability to immediately boost the function of all the five nerves required for social engagement. Revisiting the subject matter of the trapezius and sternocleidomastoid, a malfunction of the tenth cranial nerve or a lack of adequate tonus in the SCM and trapezius muscles are the causes of a lot of health issues apart from stiffness in the neck and shoulders. These health issues include difficulty in breathing, severe dorsal vagal state, reduced life expectancy, acute spinal sympathetic chain activation, forward head posture, and migraine.

Also, in determining the shape and health of the spine, the trapezius and SCM play a crucial role. In addition, severe tension in the SCM muscles on one side has the ability to change the shape of the back of the head. When this occurs, it leaves the back of the head flat on one side because of the continuous pull of the muscle on the skull plates behind the ears. An instance of this had been seen in every child that has been treated for autism spectrum. In each of them, it was observed that, there is a distortion in the shape of the back of the head.

The act of turning the head to either side should be a seamless and coordinated activity that should be done without stops, jerks, and deviation from a smooth curve. Typically, the head should be able to turn slightly more than ninety degrees. Often, people complain about the reduction in movement, pain, and stiffness in their neck and shoulders when they turn their head to one side. The shoulder problem is most likely to be either of the trapezius or the SCM on the side toward which they are turning if the pain is on the side opposite to the direction in which they turn their head. However, if the pain is on the same side as the turn, the problem is not the eleventh cranial and the trapezius and SCM but is most likely due to the levator scapulae. The exercise that can improve the neck's capacity for lateral movement is called the Salamander exercise. It could be painful at first. However, if one is persistent, the range of motion of the neck could be increased. In addition, the flow of blood to the eleventh cranial nerve could be improved. The function of the trapezius and SCM could be improved.

The Levator Scapulae Muscle

The Basic Exercise and the Salamander exercises can improve the function of the cranial nerves. It could also enhance the rotation of the head to the right and left. However, these might not be enough to allow full freedom in the turning of the head, since many other muscles of the neck are involved in the head movement and tension in any of them can hinder the turning of the head.

For instance, if we have a pain in our neck on the same side our neck is turning to, then the problem is not the eleventh cranial nerve, the trapezium, and SCM. The most likely reason is that it is coming from the levator scapulae. In these cases, working on the eleventh cranial nerve, the trapezium, and the SCM will most likely not remove all the pain and stiffness. It has been discovered that directly massaging the levator scapulae gives temporary relief. This is because the dysfunction of the muscle returns quickly. This is because the levator scapulae are an undertone. This is why it is recommended. In order to get a lasting result, it is suggested that one should massage the supraspinatus.

The Trapezius and Sternocleidomastoid muscles

Issues with the trapezium and the sternocleidomastoid muscles are more severe than the discomforts of pain, migraines, or stiffness. Most times, people with a malfunction of either the trapezius or the sternocleidomastoid muscles are not socially engaged. Also, they are susceptible to all of the issues earlier described in the "head of the hydra case." Amending the function of these two muscles usually boosts the role of the eleventh cranial nerve and can reinstate the state of social engagement. Since these are innervated by a cranial nerve, they are diverse 660 skeletal muscles in the rest of the body, which are innervated by the cranial nerves. Tautness in any of these muscles can cause pain, stiffness, and reduced movement. Malfunction in the sternocleidomastoid and trapezius muscles, by disparity, is related to a host of severe health issues that are not usually associated with muscular problems.

The trapezius muscles are a duo of thin, flat, trapezoid-shaped, superficial muscles that cover a large of the back of the neck, torso, and shoulders. They stem from the occipital bone at the base of the back of the skull. Also, they are attached to the spinous processes of each vertebra of the cervical and thoracic spine and the shoulder blade. The SCM muscles attach to the tip of the mastoid process of the temporal bones, along with the skull behind the ears. The muscle then splits into two parts that wrap diagonally forward and down. Also, one-part attaches to the top of the breastbone and the other part to the middle of the collarbone. Since the two muscle parts attach at slightly different places on the skull and they pull the head at slightly different angles. In addition, since the sternal and clavicular parts of the SCM attach in various locations on the torso, they also contribute to the rotation of the head.

The sternocleidomastoid muscles on both sides can be equated to reins that allow a horse rider to control the way his horse head moves. The horse rider pulls in the reins on one side while letting slack on the other side. If the tension in the SCM is not severe on either side, our head would be balanced correctly on our neck, and it would turn quickly to the right or left without hindrance or pain. Also, the head would come to a natural resting position looking straight ahead.

On the flip side, most times, there is usually tightness in one of the parts of the SCM on one side. This results in a stiff neck. By this, the rotation of the neck accessible toward one side but delicate on the other. Since the sternocleidomastoid is innervated by the CN XI, this stiffness is most times caused by a malfunction of the eleventh nerve and is almost always the same with a breakdown of the vagus nerve.

If the parts of the SCM that are attached to the sternum tighten symmetrically on both sides, they will shorten the neck, making it thicker. By this, they will pull the head forward. This has been described as a "bull neck." If the parts of the sternocleidomastoid that are attached to the clavicle tighten symmetrically, they pull the head backward, making the neck what s described a swan neck.

One of the works of a very popular body therapist calls our attention to the fact that the trapezius and the SCM encompass the outering of muscles of the neck. Inside this, there are many muscles that are smaller and help our heads to move better, to lift the upper ribs, and to swallow. The intricate coordination of tension and relaxation muscles that turn the head requires precise muscle control. This is set into our nervous system in such a way that we do not have to think about the procedure of it. For instance, when something catches our fancy, we automatically concentrate on it. Our head then moves in the direction of our eyes, and our body follows suit. The eyes focus on an object of interest and center it in the visual field. Afterward, the CN XI innervates the fibers of the SCM and trapezius muscles in order to turn the head in that direction. It is a fact that from birth, we have the unique ability to coordinate the movement of our eyes, body, and head. For instance, when a boy is lying on his stomach, and an object in front of him moves or changes speed, his eyes will focus on the purpose and follow the movement with his eyes and his head. As grown-ups, we respond in the same way. If a sound catches our attention, we move our head to center the sound between or eyes. This process requires intricate coordination of the trapezius, SCM, and other muscles.

The Serengeti Plain: The Trapezius and SCM muscles in action

It is no news that the fastest mammal on earth is the cheetah. It is able to run at an incredible speed of up to sixty miles per hour. The cheetah does this by keeping its eyes fixed on the prey it is aiming at. The CN XI equips the cheetah to turn its head, and the body follows as it turns its head.

A prey like an antelope, when chased by the cheetah, looks for a clear space where it can run to in order to escape from the cheetah without bumping into anything. When it locates such a place, its head turns in that direction, and its body follows. The antelope has an advantage, although it does not have the same speed levels as the cheetah; It has a very light body and thin legs that enable it to run faster when pursued. Also, if it runs in a straight line, it would get caught by the cheetah. By this, the antelope runs in a zig-zag front. The cheetah cannot run efficiently in this type of direction (Zigzag). By being very agile, a healthy adult antelope will escape being chased by a cheetah. Also, the antelope has a lot of endurance that makes it run for more extended periods than the cheetah that can only run at the optimal speed for a while. When any predator chases its prey for more extended periods and cannot catch it, it becomes exhausted from the intense exertion, and it takes the predator several hours to regain its strength and try again. By this, before the predator goes on a chase, it spends time to study the prey in order to pick out the one that is, newborn, old, or injured.

For the prey and predator, survival depends partly on the ability to turn the head quickly. The muscles that make this possible are the SCM and trapezium, which are innervated by the eleventh cranial nerve. Since the action of turning the head is a matter of life and death, it is not shocking that the structure of the eleventh cranial nerve is complex and intricate for accurate innervation of the fibers of these muscles.

Crawling: Function of the trapezium

The trapezium is one of the foremost muscles that babies use. When a baby lies on its stomach, the first move it takes is to arch its back and lift its head using the trapezius muscles. With its head up, it can turn its head and turn its head using the SCM. The next stage in the baby's growth is the ability to lift its head high enough to bring its head under shoulders to sustain the mass of its upper body. When this happens, the baby will soon be able to walk on all fours. At this stage, the tautness of the fibers of the upper trapezius extends and arches the neck, lifts the head and lifts the face forward. In doing this, the baby tenses all the fibers of the three parts of the trapezius equally. It arches its lower back with its lower trapezius, pulls the shoulder together with the middle trapezius, and lifts its head up and tips it back with the upper trapezius. Apart from the trapezius muscles, the head is held up and balanced on the vertebrae of the neck, partly due to the action of the largest muscle in the posterior neck. Afterward, the SCM can then rotate the head easily. At this growth stage, the baby supports its weight on its knees and hands and moves like four-legged mammals. After a while, the baby can then begin to crawl, moving its first arm forward and the other one back. This asymmetrical pattern of arm movement when crawling requires using the trapezius muscles.

By means of the body supported on all fours, the arms and thighs are at a ninety-degree angle to the trunk. By action of pushing down its arm, there is an equal force pushing the arm back up into the socket of the shoulder joint. The proprioceptive nerves in the shoulder joint can account for the brain that the arms and shoulders are balanced.

Going from Crawling to Standing: Changes that occur in the trapezium

When crawling, babies, their mass on all fours. Human beings have the same corporeal structure as four-legged animals in terms of the nerves, bones, and muscles involved in the movement. We live in a world controlled by gravity, and gravity is always pulling us down. When we were little and crawled on all fours, we shared our mass evenly on our four limbs, which held our mass by pushing up into our body.

When we grew and stood on our hind legs to balance, we had to use our muscles and bones in away. The dynamics of the tension in our muscular and skeletal systems changed. Instead of even muscle tonus in the fibers of the muscles, some muscles became severely taut, and others became limp. Rather than support our weight on all fours, we balance our heavy body on the two ball and socket joints between the hips and legs when we stand. This is a better way of standing than crawling on all fours.

As time goes on, standing on our back legs can cause problems that four-legged animals do not have. The most common one is an increase in our forward head posture. This happens as we advance in age. At the stage of crawling on all fours, the trapezius muscles held our head up high. The three parts of the trapezium functioned as a single muscle in which all the fibers had nearly the same tension. Some muscles worked together to pull the shoulders back and together in order to provide support for the upper spine. Other muscle fibers, pulling in different directions, had the function of lifting the head back up. However, when we began to stand, some part of the trapezium lost their viability as they were no longer needed to pull or shoulders together in the back and tilt our head up. Instead of acting as one muscle, these muscle fibers divided themselves into three viable units. These units are now known as the upper, middle, and lower trapezius. These three functional units began to work as separate units. By this, one part might be very taut while the other is not. This shows in the position of not only the bones of the shoulder but the spine too.

A humans' spine is much different from that of the goat, sheep, giraffe, or horse. A typical four-legged animal supports a part of its mass by its front legs while the human beings' arms hang freely from the joint of the shoulder. At this point, there is no longer a pushing of the arms shoulder.

For instance, if we have shoulder pain, most times, we ask ourselves what we did to cause the pain; probably we lifted something substantial or did something that we are not used to. However, a factor that is not recognized in the formation of imbalances leading to shoulder pain might change that has happened because we are standing upright on our legs. Also, there is one that can tell what a lifetime habit of sitting still on chairs does to our musculoskeletal structure. This is why it is not surprising that many physical therapists report that the most common problems they treat are shoulder pains.

The spine of humans has some weaknesses that lead to stiff necks, backaches, and shoulder issues. For instance, when we stand up, the association between the head and the spine changes to when in contrast to when we were on all fours. In order to balance on our legs, the upper part of the trapezius is no longer situated to hold the head back. Also, the head tends to slide forward.

The middle part of the trapezius does not pull the shoulder blades together toward the base any longer. This is in order to make a stable base. Instead, for most of us, our shoulder blades move down our back, forward and around to our sides. In comparison to the muscular chest of a four-legged animal, our upper chest caves in, and our belly hangs out. If a person who was acting struck this posture, they would resemble someone who lost their self-esteem.

When the lower part of the trapezius does not work as it used to when we were crawling, our spine shortens, and the spine moves into a forward position. These changes are not due to increased muscular tautness but instead to a general loss of balanced tonus in the three parts of the trapezius that used to hold up our head up against the pull of gravity.

Therefore, to boost the function of the trapezius muscle, there is a need to increase the tonus of the fibers of the muscle in all the parts of the trapezius by stirring the tissue of the nerves to the muscles. This can be done by a method called the twist and turn exercise. In contrast to most exercises, this one does not stretch or strengthen the muscle. It does this by contracting and relaxing muscle tension. What it does is that it stirs up the nerves by innervating the trapezius muscle. Excessively tense areas of the muscle can relax while muscle tone increases in areas where needed.

Asymmetry in trapezius muscle tension

There are always distinctions in tension among groups of fibers. This comprises of the upper, middle, and lower trapezius muscles. Also, there is a distinction between the left and right sides. This asymmetry of the different parts can change the balance in the two shoulders. Since the trapezius is attached to the cervical and thoracic spine, disproportions in the tension between the right and left muscles of the trapezius add to rotations, flexions, side-bending, and extensions of the thoracic vertebrae. This changes the space within the chest, which then affects the function of the heart and lungs.

Asymmetry, at times, can cause can also compress the spinal nerves leaving these segments, affecting the organs they serve. Some spinal nerves go to the heart, some to the lungs, and others connect to different visceral organs.

Asymmetry in SCM tension

The sternocleidomastoid muscles on both sides are equated to primary muscles for turning the head left and right. Also, severe stress in sternocleidomastoid muscle results in a stiff neck. A baby with a stiff neck has the tendency to turn its head to one side when lying on its back. However, as the child advances in age, the condition is diagnosed as a twisted neck.

For instance, if one scrutinizes the back of the head of a person with a stiff neck, one might find it to be flat on one side. If this happens, this method described in the "method for making a flat back of head round" that will be described later in this book may not only decrease a tight sternocleidomastoid muscle but also, to some extent, start to round the back of the head.

Usually, a stiff neck goes with a rotation of the first cervical vertebra called the atlas. This results in a reduction in the flow of blood to the brainstem. In adults, a stiff neck may show a malfunction of the eleventh cranial nerve, which is one of the five cranial nerves that are needed for social engagement. Therefore, discharging SCM tension most times makes it easier for us to be socially engaged.

CN XI: A NEW PICTURE

The activity of turning the head is one of the most crucial and intricate movements of the body. It is one of the primary and first movement that a baby makes. Also, we are not strangers to this movement, and we usually do not think about it. Control of the trapezius and SCM muscles requires a matched tensing and relaxation of many individual muscle fibers. This action depends on a well-functioning eleventh nerve. Lots of anatomical illustrations depicting the eleventh cranial nerve attempt to show all the branches of this nerve in a single drawing. However, these drawings depicting the nerve have been generally confusing. It is important to note that there is a branch of the eleventh cranial nerve comes from the brainstem and is called the cranial division. Currently, it is seen as a part of the vagus nerve, the branch that innervates the pharyngeal muscles.

The spinal accessory nerve exits the spinal cord in the neck just below the cranium prior to going straight to the fibers of the trapezius and sternocleidomastoid muscles. Additionally, there is another branch of the spinal accessory nerve that consists of nerve branches that leave the spinal cord, weave together, spread into the cranium via the foramen magnum, spread across the base of the skull and exit through the jugular foramen at the floor of the skull.

Although they have different pathways, all branches of the eleventh cranial nerve work together in an organized manner to innervate the various parts of the trapezius and sternocleidomastoid muscles.

The eleventh and tenth cranial nerve has a very close affinity not only in function, through the role they play as the two of the five cranial nerves that are crucial for social engagement but structurally. A vivid link can be seen between the branches of the eleventh cranial nerve and the ventral branch of the vagus nerve after they leave the skull through the jugular foramen when they leave the jugular foramen, fibers from the eleventh cranial nerve intermix with fibers of the vagus nerve that are not within the cranium for a few millimeters. In addition to the mixing of their nerve fibers after they leave the jugular foramen, both the eleventh cranial nerve and the ventral vagus branch come from the nucleus ambiguus, a strip of nerve fibers in the brainstem. This is why it is not surprising that the normal function or malfunction as do tests for the ventral branch of the tenth cranial nerve, ventral vagus branch, and the eleventh cranial nerve.

The trap squeeze test done for the eleventh cranial nerve gives a hint of the function or malfunction of not only the eleventh cranial nerve but the other four nerves that are crucial for social engagement. The five nerves work hand in hand, and if one is deficient, the others will also have problems. Also, if the function of one of these nerves is boosted, the others will also receive a boost.

As a therapist, when you first begin to the trap squeeze for the eleventh and tenth cranial nerve function, and you ask your clients to open their mouth and say "ah-ah-ah", you would notice that whenever there is a disparity in tension between the trapezius muscles on both sides, there would be a dysfunction in the ventral vagus

If you carry out this test on eighty people starting from testing the ventral vagus with the uvular-lift filter test for vagal pharyngeal branch function and then the CN XI using the trap squeeze test. You will discover that there is a 100 percent link between the results that these two tests produce. On the basis of this, it is safe to conclude that testing the trapezius muscles is a valid 8Indicator of vagal function or malfunction.

Again, after the patient does the Basic exercise, you need to retest them using the methods you have used before. When you do this, you will notice a marked improvement in the eleventh cranial nerve and the ventral branch of the vagus nerve. You will find out that when you squeeze, the two sides seem alike. You can then ask the patients to turn their heads, and you can then explore the feelings in their shoulders, neck, and head. In most cases, you will discover that the patients will have improved movement, and they will be able to turn their head without pain.

Neck Problems and The Trap Squeeze Test for shoulder

Patients who visit body therapists and physical therapists have some common complaints. They include pain in the shoulder and stiffness of the neck. Most times, the cause of these issues consists of a lack of proper tonus of the trapezius and the SCM, either of which may be severely tense or flaccid.

Most therapists begin their treatment by working directly on tight shoulder muscles, ignoring the state of the patient's autonomous nervous system. In order to achieve the best results with myofascial release, fascial release, or release of tension in the muscles generally, it is crucial to have a ventral vagus nerve that is functioning at its optimum before trying any intervention. By this, it is advised that you first test the ventral branch of the vagus nerve or use the test that will be talked about below to test the function of the eleventh cranial nerve. This test does not take time and is less disturbing than the other test for vagal function

For this test, you only have to squeeze the muscles on the top of the shoulder. The Trap Squeeze test only takes a few seconds. Also, it is well suited for use on people and children on the autism spectrum, with whom you might encounter difficulties in getting their cooperation for the usual method.

To use this test, you must first practice it on several people in order to develop the needed kinesthetic skills. It is perfectly normal to feel unsure the first time you try testing the trapezius muscles. However, you will find that you can get the feet of it after attempting it a few times.

The eleventh cranial nerve can be verified by lifting, sliding, and rolling on top of the muscles of the trapezius and associating them on the left and right sides. The trapezius muscle is very thin, although it covers a vast area.

- First, hold the muscles of the trapezius on each side. Squeeze it lightly between your thumb and your first finger. Although, lots of therapists grab the muscle, the milder the squeeze, the better.
- If you squeeze slowly or lightly, you will be able to lift the muscles away from the underlying muscles.
- Equate the tonus of the muscle of the trapezius on one side with the tonus of the muscle of the trapezius on the other side. Examine if the two sides feel the same to you or if one side is harder than the other. Typically, the two sides should be elastic and soft. However, the usual thing is that one side is most times stretchy and soft while the

other side is not. If you squeeze with light pressure, slowly, you can feel that the muscle on one side remains soft, palpable, and relaxed if you push into it, while the other side may react if you squeeze by tensing up and feeling hard, although you may feel slight pressure.

- Ask the patient that you are testing how they feel when you squeeze the two sides; do they feel different? If the person feels different, ask the person what side is tenser? When you do this, and you and the patient discuss things, you will definitely agree that one side is harder than the other.

- When you and your patient agree that there is a difference, this is an indication that the eleventh cranial nerve is dysfunctional. This would indicate that the person's autonomous nerve is not socially engaged, and they are in a state of stress or dorsal vagal withdrawal. By this, the necessary steps can be taken to restore the ventral vagal function before moving with another therapeutic method.

Health problems connected to Forward Head Posture

Lots of health problems can come from kyphosis or forward head posture, which is connected to a malfunction of the trapezius and sternocleidomastoid muscles. Forward head posture is one result of poor posture.

As we age, a lot of us lose the good posture that we enjoyed as kids. Also, we may have increased difficulty breathing and be bothered by occasional giddiness. These problems are not considered to be medical difficulties. Also, doctors tend to assume that they are a natural part of aging and that nothing can be done about them. There is no remedy for these conditions as such.

Forward Head Position

The neck has an inclination to sag when someone has a forward head position. The upper chest collapses, reducing the space inhalation, and this results in severe breathing.

As time goes on and the forward head position gets worse, the patient tends to lose an increased portion of breathing capacity. Forward head position is most times associated with people that have breathing issues such as asthma and COPD. This is why they experienced general tiredness and decreased levels of energy. An extensive study shows that those with breathing issues have short life expectancy; shorter than those who smoke lots of cigarettes

Apart from reduced breathing capacity, the loss of internal chest space puts a lot of burden on the heart and throngs the blood vessels that go and come from the heart. The forward head position also compresses the spaces between the vertebrae of the upper thorax and neck, putting a burden on the spinal nerve on the spinal nerves of the upper thoracic spine and the neck.

Again, forward head posture compresses the vertebral arteries that convey blood to the head. This reduces blood supply to the brainstem, face, and parts of the brain, where the five cranial nerves necessary for social engagement come from. If sufficient blood circulation is not received by these nerves, they will not function well, and it is likely for one to be in a state of chronic stress

Lots of stress, aches, stiffness, and pain grow over time due to fading posture. Forward head posture results in long-term muscle strain, arthritis, pinched nerves, and herniated discs. Also, it has been stated that the loss of the cervical curve stretches the spinal cord and results in disease. The hardening of the neck in forward head posture also hardens the entire spine. Most of the stimulation and nutrition to the brain is made by the movement of the spine. On the part of emotion, they may experience disinterest and indifference about what is happening and symptoms of dorsal vagal withdrawal.

Viewing it from the side, our head should be considered directly above the middle of the shoulder. As we grow older, lots of head succumb to forward head posture. At this stage, one can see that the ear has shifted forward in relation to the center of the shoulder. This stage is usually marked by stooping over, collapsed upper chest, and imbalance of the head of the neck. The muscles of the neck have to do extra work to keep the head from tipping further forward.

Every inch of FHS can boost the mass of the head on the spine by ten pounds. The head weighs about twelve pounds, and a lot of us have our heads forward by two to three inches. FHP often results in a malfunction in the trapezius and SCM muscles. The trapezius lacks adequate tonus, while some parts of the sternocleidomastoid muscles are in severe tension. Refining the muscular tonus of these muscles restores the head back to its normal position.

Generally, there are many forms of massages and movements that work well on the body. However, since these two muscles are innervated by the cranial nerves, a different approach is used on them. The first step in restoring normalcy in either of the two muscles is doing the Basic Exercise. Most times, when a client does this exercise, it helps in restoring the head partly to its former position. In order to improve FHP further and bring the head back to the normal position, it is advised to use the salamander exercise and the Twist and turn exercise

FHP: The contribution of Scar tissue

Most of the time, scar tissues are formed after surgery in order to fortify the body against the occurrence of a similar wound at the same place. It is possible for the patient to know that this extra tissue is unnecessary because there is a slim likelihood that an incision will be made at the same place next time, but the connective tissue does not know this.

In truth, the surgery might have been life-saving. However, the folds of muscle and fascia bind together as then incision heals. This contraction in the fascial network spreads beyond where the incision was initially made to affect the whole body. It is a fact that every surgery has its negative aspect, which is always glossed over.

Although the scar tissue may not be visible on the surface, there could be an extensive buildup of scar tissue in the linking muscles under the skin and in deeper areas. Although the surgery might have been done to minimize the scars, scar tissue still spread to other areas.

Ideally, there should be an amount of thick fluid between adjacent layers of muscle and connective tissue; this allows them to slide freely across each other. However, during surgery, this fluid may drain out, causing those tissues to begin to stick together. In addition, after surgery, the connective tissue produces more collagen fibers that can connect one layer of muscle to another. When two layers have stuck together, they can no longer slide across each other like before. Lots of surgeons are always meticulous in making sure that each layer of tissue is sewn together without sewing other tissues together.

Sadly, some surgeons do not understand the need to be meticulous in this case and might sew layers together without paying attention to detail in order to save time and money. The consequence is that the muscles become less flexible in that area. For instance, if the scar tissue is from a C-section, the scar goes all the way from the skin surface to the uterus; In case it is the abdomen, the scar tissue hinders the space for breathing. After surgery, the individual layers dry out and stick together, thereby hindering movement. Connective tissue in front of the body tightens and shortens the front of the body and pulls the head further down. This is why it is recommended that anyone who has abdominal or chest surgery to find a massage therapist who is experienced and skilled in freeing tensions from the scar tissue.

The concept of the treatment of scar tissue is couched on the desire to work on restrictions in individual layers of muscle and connective tissue. Also, it is centered around freeing the different layers from each other so that one layer can slide feeling on the adjoining layer. It is a fantastic thing when one looks at the rate of improvement that occurs in the motion in the neck, spine flexibility, and posture improvement after releasing the scar tissue.

Suboccipital muscle tension and FHP

The fine-tuning of the movements of the muscles in the head and neck comes from the small suboccipital muscle located between the occiput and the two vertebrae of the neck, whereas the SCM and trapezius provide massive rotational movement of the head and neck. Three of these muscles are what is made up of a place called the suboccipital triangle. The pressure is put on the suboccipital nerve and the vertebral arteries nearby, which are rooted in the connective tissue of the suboccipital triangle when the suboccipital muscles are taut. The implication of this is a reduction of blood supply to the brainstem and the five cranial nerves that are crucial for social engagement. With FHP, the muscles of the suboccipital triangle tauten in order to keep the chin from falling forward onto the chest. When these muscles are kept in a state of constant contraction, they contract further. This accentuates the FHP more and can cut down the flow of blood to the brainstem. This is why it is not shocking that most people with FHP often complain of headaches at the back of their head, under the base of the cranium where the suboccipital muscles are located. When pressure is applied on the suboccipital muscles, it could express itself as pain at the back of the neck. In some patients, they complain that they feel as though they are not getting enough blood flow to their heads.

It has been observed that patients with asthma have a poor ventral vagal function. Most times, they always have a forward head posture. Also, they have a stiff upper thoracic spine and reduced the lateral expansion of their chest when breathing in. Reducing the condition improves their breathing.

Usually, the Basic Exercise releases the tension in the suboccipital muscles. The first cranial nerve rotates back into place, pressure on the vertebral arteries is reduced, the blood flow to the brainstem is increased, and this improves the capacity for social management.

Relieving Migraine Headaches

COPD migraines do not take years off one's life expectancy, but they reduce the quality of one's life. There are many drugs for migraines, but they do not work all the time for everyone; some medicines are expensive, and they have side effects. However, lots of people want to be free from medications altogether. Twenty-eight million people in the United States suffer from migraines. Migraine headaches are one of the costliest health problems in terms of time lost from work. Migraine headaches, mostly called tension headaches, differ from moderate to severe and are most times sharp and throbbing. The maximum number of days it spans is three days, and they occur with signs of automatic dysfunction. They could come suddenly and go suddenly.

Typically, Migraines could come with other signs such as

nausea, vomiting, fatigue, oversensitivity to light, blurred vision, visual distortions, and dizziness. For women, it might come in the form of headaches at a particular point in their menstrual cycle.

Most times, doctors classify migraines into different types. This depends on the accompanying symptoms, and patients usually want to give thorough information about these signs, including how long ago the headache started and how long they last. Although the information is crucial to the patient, it does not help as a therapist to treat them.

It is a fact that if the migraines can be cured, the symptoms can be gotten rid of. In order to treat migraine effectively, it is essential to know the side of the head that the migraine is on and which two muscles of the neck are involved.

As a therapist, in order to show this, it is advised to confirm your client's visual examples. This could be in the form of four drawings of the trapezius and sternocleidomastoid muscle. The red areas in the drawings illustrate the patterns of pain that can come. Typically, the migraine sufferer is asked to pick out which side of the head the pain appears, and which parts of the two major neck muscles are involved.

When this is done, you will discover that they will be able to identify which of these drawings shows their pattern of pain. With this information, you will know which muscle is involved. Primarily, a therapist should be concerned about the pattern of the pain, which would tell you exactly where you should intervene with your hands. You can find the different patterns of tension causing these headaches, where to manage specifically for each pattern.

A prominent therapist by the name Dr. Janet Travell was able to relieve President Kennedy of the severe back pains he suffered from his time in the Navy in World War II. Dr. Travell's research shows that tautness in individual muscles brings about specific patterns of pain. Lots of inexperienced massage therapists just massage where it hurts. However, muscle tension often produces pain and other symptoms in other parts of the body. Referred pain is described as pain at a distance from the source of the pressure. She found that treating specific points in muscles not only relieves pains close to those points that can reduce referred pains. She called it "trigger points."

Trigger points are found in all muscles. The therapist has to observe that they feel a little harder as compared to other areas on the exterior of the muscle. The patient will also feel that those points are painful. Massaging trigger points release the pain in the area locally. Also, it relives referred to pain occurring at a distance from tense muscles. Releasing tension in the trapezius and sternocleidomastoid muscle of the neck by pressing the proper trigger points, relieves migraine headaches.

Biomechanical craniosacral therapy gives specific methods to free blockages to the CN XI at the point where it leaves the cranium. The best results are gotten when you improve the function of the eleventh cranial nerve before releasing tension in the muscles with light pressure on the trigger points. Relief from migraines is faster and long-lasting. Lots of patients are shocked to feel relief on the very first treatment.

If the CN XI is dysfunctional, the ventral branch of the vagus nerve and the CN IX are usually malfunctioning as well. Treatment of the three nerves instantly improves the function of the other two so that you do not treat the three nerves one at a time. Usually, the Basic Exercise makes the three nerves functional. Some schools of thought on the subject of migraine believe that the major causes of migraines are unknown. By this, it makes migraines hard to treat. Extensive studies demonstrate that some emotional conditions could be linked to migraines, including the activity of the dorsal branch of the vagus, bipolar disorder, and anxiety.

These pertinent questions need to be asked, do migraines have a musculoskeletal component? Over the years, it has been discovered over the years that boosting the function of the tenth cranial nerve and eleventh cranial nerve, followed by releasing the tautness in these muscles using.

Chapter 9: Somatopsychological Issues

Many years ago, orthodox doctors started dragonizing some health as problems that relate to the fact that the mind causes issues in the body. However, extensive research has shown the reverse of the case.

Psychology comes from the earliest Greek meaning study of the mind. Currently, describing a problem as psychological means that a psychologist searches for the solution in the spirit of the clients using verbal therapy.

Note that in this ancient definition, the body was not mentioned. When psychoanalysis pioneered by Feud started to help people with their psychological issues, the method of his treatment was strictly verbal. In this approach, he allowed people to talk, and he listened intently. Also, there was a dialogue; neither was there any eye contact. People had psychoanalysis for years often going to many sessions per week.

By training, a psychiatrist must be a medical doctor. They go through their process of psychoanalysis, which could take lots of years. At a point, there were few psychiatrists, and people could not afford them. Psychologists mapped out a new outline that was different from that of ancient psychologists. In the university system, psychologists are trained over a few years. They rely on various models to help their patients and into a dialogue with them using several verbal approaches. Generally, they are looking for solutions to specific problems. Psychological treatment is still expensive, although not as expensive as psychoanalysis.

Group therapy is offered by some therapists, and it is less expensive because many patients share the cost of a session. Currently, we are swiftly moving away from these measures and relying on prescription drugs to change our behaviors. After professional consultation to select the medicine and dosage, patients can go for an extensive period of time using their medications without needing to visit a doctor. Although prescription drugs could be costly, they are efficient when compared to ongoing one-on-one healing processes with mental health professionals. However, because more people take these medications, this type of treatment is tantamount to a growing expense for the patient as well as for the Insurance companies and the economy of the nation.

Since Psychiatry and psychology began with a sole emphasis on the mind and because of the widespread availability and use of prescription and use of prescription medicines, we could be missing out on another thing that could help us with these health problems that these prescription medicines aim to address. Maybe there is something at our fingertips that has no side effects.

This is why, in this chapter, we will take an in-depth look into how we could use bodily exercises to correct mental and emotional issues. Also, we will look into how self-help exercises and hands-on methods can be totally safe and active in achieving the best of changes. Through research, it is believed that the in-depth knowledge of the polyvagal theory can help us to treat our own autonomic nervous systems. It just might be possible for us to overcome what has been prior to this time seen as untraceable psychological and psychiatric issues.

The autonomous nervous system and Emotions

Before we begin, let us ask ourselves, are we shut down, depressed, or apathetic? Are we angry, aggressive, fearful, or withdrawn? Are we open., friendly, communicative, and cooperative? How do we react to other people when we are in these states?

Other people's response to us is based on a blend of the state we are in and the state they are in. Emotions play a significant role in the relation between the states of our autonomous nervous system and theirs.

We are social animals and mammals. By this, we need others. We all encounter challenges and doubt occasionally. In order to increase our chances for survival and accomplishment, we depend on our contact with others; friends, family, social network, and neighbors. Our feelings in a situation or about someone is a factor that determines how we behave.

The proper function of the social engagement cranial nerves is crucial to how we communicate and bond with others. These five nerves aid our hearing, shape the sounds of our speech, and help us understand what other people mean.

The autonomous nervous system and emotional states are seen as two sides of a coin. If we want to boost our emotional state in order to help ourselves or others, we can do this with physical actions that improve the state of our autonomous nervous system and move us out of a stress state into social engagement.

The autonomous nervous system: A self-regulating one

Personal contact with people who are in a state of social engagement and balance is possibly the most natural and effective way to achieve self-regulation. In the instance of encountering a problem, it is not enough to talk about it with just a friend or trusted relative.

Chapter 10: Drills to Reinstate Social Engagement

T his part is targeted at going through the healing power of the tenth cranial nerve. Top-notch health is a possibility when the ventral branch of the vagus nerve is functioning at the optimum. The drills and methods will help a lot of people to move from a state of severe stress or shutdown to a state of social engagement. In addition, these methods could be used to avert issues in the autonomic nervous system from growing. Also, it helps to maintain a general level of well-being.

When a patient begins to engage in these drills for the first time, it is suggested that the patient starts a simple journal. The patient is advised to take down any signs or issues that disturb you. It is also recommended to look at the symbols listed in the first part of this book. Afterward, note how frequently a symptom has occurred and indicate how strong it is. After the patient has been doing these drills, you can then look back and observe the changes. Also, as a therapist, you can look at the positive and negative signs that will result from the drills. It could be that some symptoms will diminish or will become nonexistent and so on.

The Basic Exercise

The aim of these drills is to boost social engagement. It changes the position of the atlas, neck vertebra, and the axis. In addition, it increases the mobility of the neck and the spine as a whole. In addition, it boosts the way blood flows to the brainstem, where the five cranial nerves crucial for social engagement come from. This can have a god effect on the ventral branch of the vagus nerve and the other four cranial nerves.

The Basic Exercise is operative, easy to do, and easy to learn. Also, it takes a few minutes to complete it.

Before and After doing the Basic Exercise

For the patient, it is advised that first, gauge the relative freedom of your head and neck. To do this, first, rotate your neck to the right as far as it is comfortable. Afterward, turn it to the center, wait a bit, and rotate it to the left. The questions you need to ask yourself after this is; how far did I turn my head to each side? Did I experience any pain or stiffness? Was there any boost or increase in my range of movement? Did the drill reduce the level of pain?

Lots of patients that are treated are shocked to experience a boost in the range of movement as they move their head from side to side. Improved mobility of the neck comes with an increase in the way blood circulates to the brainstem. Consequentially, this boosts the function of the ventral branch of the vagus nerve.

Basic Exercise Directions

At the beginning of these drills, you should lie on your back. As time goes on and you become conversant with the drills, you can perform them while sitting, lying, or standing. These are the direction to follow when doing the Basic Exercise drills

1. While lying on your back comfortably, interlace the fingers of one hand together with the fingers of the hand.

2. Then put your hands behind the back of your head with the mass of your head resting securely on your interlaced fingers. When doing this, you must feel the stiffness of your fingers with your fingers. Also, you should feel the bones of your head. For instance, if you have a hard shoulder and have difficulty in bringing your two hands up behind the back of your head, you could use one hand with the fingers and palm, meeting both sides of the back of the head.

3. While putting your head in a fixed position, look to the right, stirring only your eyes as far as you can. Make sure it is solely your eyes, you turn and not your head. Keep looking to the right.

4. After thirty to sixty seconds, you will swallow, sigh, or yawn. This is a sign of a letup in your autonomic nervous system.

5. Bring your eyes to look ahead

6. Put your hands in place, and keep your head still. Move your eyes to the left.

7. Keep your head in place until you notice a yawn, sigh, or swallow

After completing the Basic drill, remove your hands and sit up. Afterward, gauge what you have encountered. Has there been any boost in how your neck moves? Has your breathing improved? Did you notice any improvement?

It is important to note that if you become faint when you sit or stand up, there is a probability that it is because you are relaxed when you are lying down, and your blood pressure has reduced. This is a regular thing. Typically, you need a minute or two before your blood pressure regulates and pumps more blood to the brain.

Ventral Vagus Malfunction and Cervical Vertebrae

When clients are tested, and it is discovered that there is ventral vagal dysfunction, it is observed that they have upper cervical misalignment, which is a rotation of the vertebrae and a tipping of the axis away from their optimal positions. Using the Basic drills always brings the patient back to a better alignment of the first and second cranial nerve. When they are retested, it is discovered that they have a normal ventral vagal function.

Rotation of the first and second cranial nerves can put a burden on the vertebral artery, which supplies the frontal lobes and the brainstem, where the five nerves that are crucial for social engagement come from. Form observation, it is believed that it takes only one negative thought to bring the first and second cranial nerve out of joint, affecting posture and physiology. This has been shown a number of times in some studies on advanced craniosacral practices. In this, those who study it are told to observe the position of the tutor's first cranial nerve.

The tutor then lays on his back, enabling those considering it to determine the location of the tutor's first cranial nerve by gently placing their thumbs on its sloping processes. If the first cranial nerve does not rotate, their thumbs would be almost horizontal. On the flip side, if one thumb were higher than the other, it would indicate a rotation of the vertebra.

The rotation of the first and second cranial nerve has evolutionary survival value. It puts a burden on the vertebral artery, dipping the flow of the brainstem. This affects the function of the five cranial nerves that are crucial for social engagement. It puts us into a non-ventral state, which in times of danger can aid our survival by closing down the higher functions when we have to fight or flee. If our neuroception suddenly registers signals from the environment showing that we are in danger, this change in our composition should be instant, and it is. Interestingly, although our nervous system is quick to be distressed, it takes a long time to settle down when we are safe again.

Trauma is not required to affect the first and second cranial nerve; the memory of a past event can do the same thing. Studies based on a scan of the brain in women with post-traumatic stress show a dip in the flow of blood to their brains' frontal lobes when they hear a repeat of the events that traumatize them.

One would imagine the memory of a trauma or a negative thought lead to an operational change such as a rotation of the first cranial nerve and the second cranial nerve? Ten muscles link the occipital bone beneath the skull with the first and second cranial nerve. Eight of these muscles are called suboccipital muscles, and they lie on the back of the vertebrae. Also, the rectus capitis lateralis and the rectus capitis anterior lie on the front of these two vertebrae. They are innervated by occipital nerve, located on the scalp at the back of the head. Unfitting tensions in any of these ten muscles are enough to shift and hold the first and second cranial nerve out of joint.

The transverse processes of each cervical vertebra have foramens or foramina to House passage of the vertebral arteries. Tipping of the vertebrae can put pressure on these arteries, dipping the flow of blood, as in a plastic garden hose; if you bend it, you shut off the flow of water. The volume of blood passing through these vertebral arteries depends on the position of the upper cervical vertebrae in the neck.

When the basic exercise is done, we lie with the mass of our head on our fingers. This burden is enough to stimulate the occipital nerve. This makes the muscles relax and come into balance with each other. When the Basic drill is done, the first two cervical vertebrae move into a better position relative to each other.

The first and second cranial nerves come back into place; it eases the tension on the vertebral arteries. This provides a better flow of blood to the brain and the brainstem and allows us to come back to social engagement. Sufficient supply of blood to the cranial nerves, brainstem, and the brain is crucial for the proper functioning of the bodily functions and the social nervous system.

Simultaneously, therefore, with a realignment of the first and second cranial nerve, there is relief of many of the symptoms that we earlier described as the heads of the hydra.

Why do we move our eyes in the Basic Exercise?

The Basic Exercise has to deal with the movement of the eyes since there is a direct neurological link between the eight suboccipital muscles that move our eyeballs.

We can unswervingly experience the link between the eye movement and changes in tension of the suboccipital muscles if we place a finger across the back of the head, just beneath and parallel to the lower edge of the skull. Leaving the head in place, if we move our eyes right or left, up and down, or diagonally, a light finger pressure should detect a small movement of the upper cervical vertebrae or a shift in the levels of tension in the muscles of the neck under the finger along with the movement of the eyes.

It has been observed that those who are socially engaged have a well-positioned first and second cranial nerve. Also, they have a well-functioning autonomic nervous system that is flexible and able to respond appropriately to a number of situations and states.

Social engagement is not a static state. Also, the position of the first and second cranial nerve should not stay fixed after doing the Basic Exercise. These bones move our physiological state shifts immediately. This could be in moments of happiness, fear, satisfaction, anger, or withdrawal. It could also be when our bodily state shifts among social engagement, dorsal vagal activation or spinal sympathetic chain activation.

Our autonomic nervous system constantly scans our internal and external environments. When all is well, the first and second cranial nerves come into place, and we get a sufficient flow of blood to the brainstem. When there is an activity of the spinal sympathetic chain, the first and second cranial nerves go out of position, thereby dipping the flow of blood to the source of the five cranial nerves in the brainstem and to some parts of the brain. This bodily mechanism takes us away from social engagement. Also, it enables us to react when we are challenged or in danger. This method is immediate and instinctive as it bypasses conscious thought. Most times, we are not aware of the change.

One of the cruxes of the treatment of stress and depression is to arrange the first and second cranial nerve using the Basic drill or with an effective myofascial release method. These interpositions release imbalances in the tension of the small muscles that hold the skull and the first two vertebrae in relation to each other. This changes the position of the atlas and the occiput. Enhanced alignment of the vertebrae, especially the first and second cranial nerve boosts the flow of blood to the brain and usually bring a quick improvement in the function of the five nerves that are crucial for the state of social engagement.

There are other forms of manual therapy that use high-velocity, short-thrust manipulative methods designed to put the first cranial nerve in place. However, it is better to use a milder approach. As a therapist, if you can give the body the right information with a gentle touch at the right place, the body will stabilize itself. Since we cannot put the first and second cranial nerve in place and expect them to stay that way enduringly, we should repeat balancing methods frequently or as necessary. Because there is no such thing as a fixed state of balance, it is useful to think of balancing an ongoing process.

Neuro-Fascial Release Method for Social Engagement

This method had been grown based on the understanding on the principles of biomechanical craniosacral therapy, osteopathy, and connective-tissue release. It had been used with massive success for many years, and many therapists have learned it. This technique takes less than five minutes to perform, highly effective, and requires no physical effort. It could be used on anyone else.

When can you use this Method?

The Basic Exercise is a modest self-help technique. Also, it is an easy and effective way to achieve the better function of the ventral vagus nerve. However, if you are a therapist, it might be better to use your hands than give the patient exercises to do. Also, you may want to mix the self-help drills with practical techniques.

The Neuro-fascial method can be used as a substitute for the Basic Exercise. It is expressly valuable for treating babies, children, and adults on the autism spectrum who lack the required verbal communication skills to absorb instruction about the Basic exercise when it might be hard to communicate with them and have them adhere to your guidelines. As a therapist, using this method gives you a nonverbal way of bringing about beneficial changes in another person's nervous system.

If what you do is a massage or other hands-on modalities, it is best that you practice this method or make your client do the Basic Exercise when you start the drills.

Instructions to follow when practicing the Neuro-Fascial Release Technique

If you are accustomed to doing massage, it is advised that you use your hands in a new way. This is to ensure that you achieve success with this method. First, use this method on yourself and know how to get a release before you try it on your patient. In order to achieve social engagement with this method, you must arouse reflexes in the loose connective tissue beneath the skin over the base of the skull. This balances the levels of tension in the small muscles between the bottom of the skull and the vertebrae of the neck. It will be easier to learn this method if the person is lying on his stomach so that you can easily see your fingers. It is advised that you start with one side of the back of the patient's head.

1. Place one finger on the occiput beneath the head on one side. Test the slide-ability of the skin over the bone. The skin should slide easily in one direction than the other over the bone.
2. Place the finger from the other hand at the top of the neck on the same side. If you push a little deeper, you should be able to feel the muscles. Use the finger to test the side ability of the skin over the muscles at the top of the neck. It should move

smoothly in the direction opposite to the direction that the other finger is sliding over the skull bone.

3. After testing, lighten the pressure. Let your two fingers slide in the opposite direction until you feel resistance.
4. Hold it a bit and hold that light tension. Hold on a bit till you get a sigh.
5. Release your fingers and allow the skin to come back to its normal state
6. Repeat the same process on the skin on the opposite side of the skull and the neck.

After this process, when the vagus nerve is retested, it should be functioning at the optimum. At that point, when the head is turned from left to right, there should be greater freedom of movement.

Correct use of the Neuro-Fascial Release Method

The way to succeed with applying the Neuro-fascial release method is getting the skin to slide and to stop at the first sign of resistance. Use your fingertips to link with the skin using the mildest touch possible. Afterward, slide the skin a very short distance over the underlying muscles, bones, and tendons.

This method is different from the ones used in other forms of massage, which targets the muscular system and therefore push into the body. It is advised that you take the time to read the step-by-step instructions so that you can learn to do it properly.

This effective method stretches the loose connective tissues under the skin. This connective is abundant in proprioceptive nerve endings. When you mildly slide the skin a short distance over the muscles and bones, you create little traction in this loose tissue, which is sufficient to arouse these nerves.

Slide the skin only a distance, until you feel the very first sign of resistance, and because you are working directly on the proprioceptive nerves do not need to use the force essential for most forms of massage that focus on the muscles. If unnecessary force is used after the first sign of resistance or the skin is slid too rapidly, the muscles and ligaments will tighten. No damage can be caused this way; the time for release will only take a longer time. In severe cases, you may not get the expected changes. Sometimes, you may discover that you are pushing so mildly that the other person reports that he or she cannot feel anything. This is good feedback. As you go on with the treatment, you will notice a tangible improvement in the ability of the skin to slide.

The Salamander Exercise

The salamander exercise progressively boosts the flexibility in the thoracic spine, releasing movement in the joints between the person's ribs and the sternum. This will increase the person's breathing capacity, reduce forward head movement head by bringing your head back into better alignment, and reduce an abnormal spine curvature.

Most of the fibers of the vagus nerve are afferent (sensory) fibers, which means that they bring information back from the body to the brain, while only a meager percent are motor fibers that carry instructions form the brain to the body. Some of the afferent fibers from parts of the ninth cranial nerve and the tenth cranial nerve screen the amount of oxygen and carbon dioxide in the blood; by boosting our pattern of breathing with these drills, we can tell the brain through the afferent nerves that we are safe and that our visceral organs are performing at optimum. Consequently, this brings about the ventral vagal activity.

However, we need to ask ourselves, which is more crucial? Is an inadequate breathing pattern the result of a dysfunctional or is a lack of ventral vagus function caused by feedback from a less than ideal breathing pattern? If there are tensions in the respiratory diaphragms and the muscles that move the ribs, feedback from the afferent vagal nerves controlling those movements will result in abnormal breathing. This may hinder a state of ventral vagal activity, just as restoring ventral vagal activity can advance the bodily condition; in practice, improving either one is helpful.

A forward head posture heads decrease the space in the upper chest that is available for breathing. The salamander exercises can create a space in the upper chest for both the heart and the lungs. Plummeting a forward head posture will also take the burden off the cervical vertebrae. Also, the Salamander drills relieve the strain on vertebral arteries. In addition, it can alleviate some back pains between the shoulders,

When performing the Salamander drill, you must bring your head to the same level as your entire spine. The stance is close to that of a salamander, which does not have a neck. This makes its head look like extra vertebrae at the top of the spine. Salamanders cannot flex, extend, rotate, or bend their heads separately in connection to the first vertebra at the top of the spine. Flexing, rotating, stretching, or side-bending of the head individually relating to the first vertebra of the spine, also lifting the head above the level of the spinal vertebrae are things the salamander is incapable of, things quickly done by other reptiles and mammals. This exercise is similar to the head posture of the salamander, which is done with the head in line with the spine.

Regarding the spinal movement, your head will be neither will it be down when you perform these exercises. Just like the salamander, the thoracic (the chest portion of the spine) will now side-bend better. In order to release muscular tensions between the ribs and the thoracic spine, utilizing a side-bending movement can be done. This will, in turn, add to the free movement of the ribs and boosts optimal breathing.

There is less flexibility in the thoracic spine, but an extension and flexion of the human spine, there is greater flexibility in the lumber vertebrae and the neck. However, with the performance of side-bending, the flexibility of the thoracic spine improves and increases. The achievement of side-bending unlocks the joints of the thoracic vertebrae and in turn, makes it move freely. In essence, the thoracic spine is much less flexible, but it can be made more flexible by performing the salamander exercise and in turn, leading to the freedom of movement of the ribs and optimal breathing.

The first level of this exercise is the Half Salamander Exercises. This level has three categories; the Half Salamander exercise with the eyes to the right, the Half

Salamander exercise with the eyes to the left, and the Half Salamander exercise- a variation. When going through the first level of the exercise, various steps that are to be taken as regards the category, and these steps should be followed strictly.

The first step to be taken when performing a salamander exercise as regards the first category, which is the Half Salamander exercise with eyes to the right, is to sit or stand in a comfortable position. In order for you to be able to carry out the salamander exercise with eyes to the right after you have sat or stood in a comfortable position, allow your eyes to look right without moving your head. After doing that, the following step is that you make your head continue to face forward, make your head tilt to the right in a way that your right ear will move closer to your right shoulder, and you should not lift your shoulder to meet your head. The third step required when doing the half salamander exercises is that you must hold your head in the position that has been stipulated by step two for thirty to sixty seconds. After holding your head in the area for at least thirty seconds, you then allow your head to come back up to neutral, and you shift your eyes to look forward.

Regarding the second category, which is the Half Salamander exercise with eyes to the left, you will repeat the same process for the left side as well. This simply means that after sitting or standing comfortably, you will allow your eyes to move left without moving your head, then you will side-bend your head to the left, staying like that for thirty to sixty minutes after which you return your head back to its upright position, and make your eyes face the forward direction.

Now, regarding the third category, i.e., Half Salamander – a variation, it is the same instructions that should be followed. However, the only discrepancy is that your eyes will look to the right while your head is tilting to the left. The benefit of this movement of your eyes before moving your head is that it increases your range of motion. Another discrepancy is that Half Salamander exercise- a variation is done for both sides. You are to hold the variation position for like thirty to sixty minutes on a side before you switch to the other side.

The second level of this exercise is Full Salamander exercise. This level has to do with the whole side-bending of the spine rather than just the neck. The full salamander exercise involves the use of body positioning. They include;

Salamander on All Fours:

This requires you supporting your body weight on your knees and your palms. In doing this, you can put your palm on the floor to give support to your body weight, but putting your palms on what will propel them up like a table, sofa, pillow, desktop, among other things, will be better. The reason why it is called Salamander on all four; a salamander is a reptile, and most reptiles walk on four legs. So, your position here will be imitating the natural mien of the Salamander.

In performing this exercise, the ears should not be dropped below or raised above the level of the spine; your position must make your head relative to your spine. To be able to get this position, lift your head slightly above what you think to be the right position, then lower your head slightly below what you think is the correct position. Doing these, you should be able to sense that your head is somewhat raised than the normal position, and your head is lower than the normal position. Then, get the position that is in between the two positions. Remember, you are still on all fours, i.e., on your palms and knees.

Once this position that makes your head relative to your spine is found, look with your eyes to the right, hold them in that position then, side-bend your head to the right making your right ear move towards your right shoulder. Allow the bending in your side to continue further than the neck, down to the base of your spine. Make sure you are in this position for thirty to sixty seconds. Afterward, bring your spine and head back to the center. This will all be done on your palms, and your knees, like how the salamander reptile look at what it is curious about.

Salamander with the Head to the left:

For this position, all the steps for Salamander on all Fours are to be repeated. However, the difference is that the steps should be carried out on the left side this time. This means you support your body weight with your palms and knees; then, you find a position that makes your head relative to your spine. When you find this position, look with your eyes to the left, hold the position, then side-bend your head to the left, making your right ear move towards your right shoulder. This side-bending should continue beyond the neck down to the base of the spine. Once in this position, hold it for like thirty to sixty minutes before you bring your head and your spine back to the center position.

These are the steps to be taken when performing the Salamander Exercise. When these steps are followed, the thoracic spine becomes more flexible, which in turn leads to optimal breathing and free movement of the ribs.

Massage for Migraine

Migraine headache pain has four different pattern illustrations. In some drawings, the location of trigger points on the surface of the muscles that can be massaged in order to release tension in the affected muscles is indicated. These drawings show the four typical patterns of migraine pain. Look for the model that best fits the symptoms of your migraine; this will make it easier to identify the part of the muscle, which is tight and where to massage it.

In these drawings, each pattern has trigger points that have been marked. The trigger points are areas on the surface of a muscle where there is a high concentration of nerve endings. These trigger points are sometimes more thick or hard than other muscles, and those that are often found to be released are painful when pressure is applied on them.

Locating and Neutralizing Tension in Trigger Points

Most humans work on nerves on the surface of the muscle, so a gentle touch is enough to release tension in the entire muscle. It is usually sufficient to massage trigger points rather than massage the whole muscle, just like in a simple massage.

When the body is under great pressure, it doesn't feel safe, and the nervous system is automatically put in a state of dorsal vagal withdrawal or sympathetic activation, and it takes the body a whole lot of time to settle down again. So, using lots of force or deep massage of trigger points is often painful and may be counterproductive. It may not be injurious, but it is ineffective.

Whenever release from a migraine headache is needed, for less pain, make a few small circles on the trigger points, stop and wait for a nervous system reaction in the form of either a sigh or a swallow. Within a few minutes, the intensity of the will starts to reduce and eventually disappear. This treatment can be repeated.

Not all the marked trigger point in the different drawing illustration of the pattern of migraine headache needs to be treated. It will be a waste of time to try to release all trigger points that have been marked on these various patterns that we have because not all of them are active and are in need of immediate release. In essence, even if the trigger point has been identified for a particular pattern of pain, if no pain or thickness or hardness is felt on its particular spot on the surface, the trigger point is not active. Disregard the non-active trigger points and focus more on the ones that are hard, thick, or painful when little pressure is applied.

SCM Exercise for Stiff Neck

By doing this exercise, your range of movement will be extended as you rotate your head, the symptoms of the stiff neck will be alleviated and prevents migraine headaches. The movement in this exercise is akin to the movement of infants, which includes lying on the stomachs, propped by the elbow with the head free to survey the surrounding. The steps required in doing this exercise include;

- Lying on the stomach, lifting the head and bringing the arms under the chest, which puts the weight of the upper body on the elbows.

- Rotating the head to head to the right as far as it can comfortably go.

- Holding that position for thirty to sixty seconds.

- Bringing the head back to the center.

- Afterward, rotating the head to the left as it can comfortably go.

- Holding that position for like thirty to sixty seconds.

- Then, bringing the head back to the center.

When you have improved the rotation of the head by doing this exercise, but you are still feeling constraints, and the movement of the head is not as good as you want it to be on one side or both sides, perhaps the restriction is coming from a different muscle, i.e., the Levator Scapulae which is innervated by spinal nerves C3-C5.

With the limitation coming from this different muscle, this stiff neck cannot be eliminated by a minor improvement of the function of the CN XI, the sternocleidomastoid and trapezius muscles. Part of the stiffness may also be from the shortening of the esophagus and a hiatal hernia because the vagus nerve wraps around the throat.

Twist and Turn Exercise for the Trapezius

This exercise helps in improving the tone of a flaccid trapezius as well as balancing its three parts with the other two parts. It aids also includes improvement in breathing, lengthening the spine, and correcting forward head posture (FHP), which in turn alleviates back and shoulder pains. The exercise which requires less than a minute to do it is not only for FHPs; it can benefit anyone. When the exercise is done, the effect is positive and instantaneous. Doing this exercise has helped me many times. I always do this position after standing up from sitting at my computer or from reading a book. It is advisable to do this exercise and repeat it many times whenever you've been sitting for a while. You will experience an improvement in posture and breathing whenever you perform this exercise. And the changes are effective and immediate. The usual assumption is that the muscle is strong enough, and it just needs to stimulate the nerves to the soft muscle fibers. So, the exercise is neither to strengthen the trapezius muscle nor to stretch them. The exercise is to awaken them so that they can complete their tasks, which they performed when we were babies when we were crawling on all fours. The baby, when lying down, uses all the fibers of the three parts of the trapezius muscles to keep the shoulder blades together; it will lift its head to turn around. The baby also uses all these muscles to raise itself up on the palms and knees to look around. The exercise takes the position of that of a crawling baby. But when the baby stands up, the trapezius muscles are not being evenly used, this makes some of them become tense, and energy goes out of the others, and they become flaccid. Since the head is no longer supported by all the three parts of the trapezius muscle, it tends to slide forward, which makes the center of the ears stay in front of the center of the shoulder. This causes the shoulder to posit the proclivity to pull forward and down towards the midline.

When you are done with this exercise, the fibers of the three parts of the trapezius will become more toned. If you stand or sit after this exercise, your head will glide back to his normal, natural position itself, increasing the posture and reducing FHP.

Instructions for the Twist and Turns Exercise

This exercise has three fragments. They are similar positions. However, the discrepancies between these parts are the positioning of the arm. You are to sit comfortably on a surface that is firm like a chair or a bench, and you keep your face looking forward. You are to fold and cross your arm; then, you rest your hands to rest lightly on your elbow. Afterward, you will rotate your shoulder girdle quickly from a side to the other without stopping and fluctuating your hips. These parts include;

- Letting your elbows drop and rest it in front of your body. Afterward, you rotate your shoulders so that your elbows will move from one side to another. When doing this; your arm girdle glides lightly over your stomach, which in turn activates the fibers of your upper trapezius. Perform these three times. Make sure you do not stop your movement and do not strain yourself. Your movement will be more relaxed and easier if you move your shoulder without forcing them or holding them.

- This part is similar to the first part; however, you have to lift your elbows and hold them in front of your chest at the heart region level. Then, rotate your elbow to a side to the other. Perform this part three times, and in turn, it activates the muscle fibers of your middle trapezius.

- You then raise your elbows high in the most comfortable manner you can and then repeat the exercise that has been stipulated. Afterward, rotate your elbows from one side to the other. Do these three times, and like the other parts, it activates the muscle fibers of your lower trapezius.

Once you are done with this part of the exercise, your head will move back and up away from the forward head posture to its original position, and your head will feel lighter. And it is okay for someone with a pronounced FHP to become a little bit taller after they have done the exercise.

A Four Minute Natural Facelift (First Phase)

This treatment makes the facial muscles to relax, improves the functions of the cranial nerves V and VII. The following are the benefits of this treatment:

- The treatment brings about a youthful liveliness.

- Between the corners of the mouth and the corners of the eyes, this treatment helps to put life in the muscles of expression.

- This treatment makes very high cheeks a little flatter and brings out flat cheekbones.

- This treatment increases the circulation of blood to the skin of the face.

- The treatment increases your sense of empathy by making your face responsive to interactions with others.

- It helps to smile often and more naturally.

- It improves the circulation of the skin.

The person trying to do this technique must be able to see a clear reflection of themselves. If you are doing it for yourself, hold a mirror to your face. If you are doing it on another person, give the person to hold the mirror to his face so that the face can be watched, and the changes can be followed. Also, take important notice of the skin around the cheekbone. It is advisable to do one side of the face first to be able to compare the two sides. The differences should become more apparent when you talk or smile.

There is a point on the face called the Golden Bamboo in Classical Thai Massage. It is a point on the face that us the endpoint of the large Intestine acupuncture meridian called the LI 20. In traditional Chinese Medicine, it is regarded as a Welcoming Fragrance because it opens the nostril, which increases and improves breathing. This point is called the Beauty point in the Chinese, Japanese, and Thai massage. This point lies over the joint directly between two bones of the face: the maxilla and the premaxilla. In modern anatomy, these bones, the maxilla, and pre-maxilla are referred to as one the maxilla. They were separated before in the evolutionary development of our species. A slight touch of the skin about an eighth of an inch to the side of the supra-alar crease, which is the fold between the cheek and the upper lip near the outer edge of the nostril, will disclose the location of the endpoint of LI 20 easily. If the supra-alar crease area is explored with the finger, the point would be easily found because it is more sensitive to the surrounding skin.

Why and How to Perform the Four Minutes Natural Facelift Treatment

There are two main areas where treatment is to be performed. On the facial skin and on the facial muscles.

The facial skin surface is innervated by branches of the fifth cranial nerve, and a light touch of the skin on the face stimulates these nerve endings. The following are the steps to be carried to do the treatment as regards the facial skin:

- At the acupuncture point, LI20, with very light contact, brush the surface of the skin. Afterward, make your fingertips melt together with the skin.

- Find the direction that posits greater resistance by sliding the skin up and down. Once found, push lightly into the resistance with the fingertips.

- Hold at the point until you feel the resistance release.

- Also, slide the skin inward towards the midline of the face and outward towards the side to find the point of greater resistance.

- Once found, push lightly into the resistance with the fingertip and hold until you feel the resistance released.

It of importance to also know that the muscles of the face are innervated by the branches if the seventh cranial nerve VII. The facial muscles have two lawyers just beneath the skin. So, as regards treatment for the facial muscles, the following steps are to be carried out:

- Sink your fingertips gently into the muscle layers below the skin at the same point. Then, make the fingertip adhere to the muscle layers.

- Be fastidious in pushing the skin. If you are careful enough not to push too hard, you begin to feel it under the fingertips, and then you can slide into these layers of the muscles gently. Then slide one layer on the top of the other, making a small circle.

- Now use your fingertips to go around the circle. While doing this, you might notice that there is more resistance to sliding the skin in one direction. Once you get this direction, keep sliding at it lightly until you feel a release that may come in the form of a swallow a sigh.

- Afterward, you will have to deal with the deeper layer of the muscles. The deeper layers of the muscles stick together with the skin and the top muscle layer. You push slightly deeper into the deeper layers of the muscle. Slide the two layers together on the surface of the bone.

It should also be known that all bones have a connective tissue covering called a periosteum, which means around the bone. This tissue is very rich in nerve endings like the cranial nerves we are talking about. This bone is another part where the treatment must touch. And the steps of treating this bone are:

- Making your fingertips sink deeper into the face until it touches and rests on the surface of the bone, i.e., the periosteum.

- Press slightly in a way that will make your fingertips reach the surface of the bone at Large Intestine 20. Then, make your fingertips form a pattern of movement on the surface of the bone. Then, just like others, mildly hold until you feel a release. The effect of massaging the surface of the periosteum is great on the automatic nervous system.

Massaging the cranial nerves V and VII stimulate the nerves to the skin and muscles of the face. It relaxes the muscles on the face, relaxes, and reduces some wrinkles leaving the face younger and refreshed; however, it doesn't remove wrinkles. A light stroking (massage) of the skin on the face stimulates CNV, which in turn reduces tension in all the facial muscles. It is an effective treatment with no side effects like toxic accumulations, scar tissues, among others. It is a great treatment for the face, which makes the face of the patient younger, lively, and restored. Furthermore, this massage treatment makes a face more socially engaged, communicative, expressive, and responsive. In addition, facial expressions are requisite when communicating with others; it is important for our faces to be able to express emotional responses to every situation. Micro-movements are automatically made by our face that mirrors the facial expression of others when our face is looking at someone else's face and is relaxed. The micro-movements are small, and they alter fast. These movements cause changes in the tension in our skins and facial muscles, which is carried to the brain through the cranial nerves V and VII that gives us the immediate information about how and what others are feeling. This is the requirement for having empathy for another person.

A person has a pleasant, smooth, and what is called beautiful or handsome face if the facial muscles are relaxed. If the facial muscles are not relaxed, they pull on the skin, which in turn creates double chin or wrinkles, and with time, the wrinkles become deeper.

Four Minute Natural Facelift (Phase Two)

Phase one of this treatment is focused on the acupuncture point on the large intestine meridian, which is at the side of the nostril, i.e., the LI 20. And as it has been explained, the stimulation of this point increases the tone and the balance of the muscles of the lower face around the mouth and nose. This second phase of the natural facelift treatment will be focusing more on the eyes. The technique for this second phase is similar to that of the first phase. The acupuncture point B2 for the second phase of this treatment is located in the inside corner of the eyebrows. When people are tired, they tend to rub this spot naturally without even thinking about it because massaging this spot, which people often do even without the thought of this treatment is self-comforting. Connect your thumb or any finger with the acupuncture point B2, then go down to each of the layers of the skin, two layers of the muscle, and the periosteum.

Massage of the B2 Acupuncture point

Like the LI 20, the B2 is also a trigger point. It is a trigger point for the orbicularis oculi muscle, which is a flat muscle that surrounds the opening of the eyes. Before the treatment of the B2, the eyes may undertone, leaving it too open, or the muscles may be too tight, which makes the eyes slightly closed. After the treatment, the balance between looking outward and looking inwards will improve, which in turn will allow you to see other people clearly.

If you go deeper, you will figure that the acupuncture point B2 is at the edge of a tiny facial bone, and this bone is called the Lacrimal bone. You can balance the moisture of the eyes and leave the eyes bright and sparkling by touching and holding this lacrimal bone at the B2 trigger point. The following are the steps to be taken in the treatment of the acupuncture point B2:

- First, find the more sensitive place than the surrounding areas at the inner corners of the eyebrows.

- Then, brush the skin lightly for a few times using your fingertips.

- Afterward, allow your fingertips to rest on the skin at the acupuncture point B2 lightly.

- Hold the contact with the surface of the skin, leaving it there till the resistance is released in the form of a swallow or a sigh.

- Next, gently press down to the layer of the facial muscle, where the orbicularis oculi muscle that goes around the eyes joins with the facial bone.

- Then, make a small circle by letting the skin stick with your finger, thus sliding the skin lightly and searching for where there is resistance.

- Once the resistance is found, hold on it till you get a release that could come in the form of a sigh or swallow.

- After this has been done, go deeper, do not stop until you make contact with the surface of the bone which you rub a few times with your fingertips.

- If a contact has been made, hold o it with the bone and wait for a release in the form of a sigh or swallow.

If the eyes were gaping, this treatment technique will bring it down a little and still leave the eyes open. If the orbicularis oculi muscle is too tight, it closes the eyelids to a squint. But with the performance of this technique, the eyes would open normally.

The main aim of these hand treatment techniques and self-help exercises is to bring people to a ventral vagal state and bring them out of a dorsal vagal state or the long-lasting activation of the sympathetic chain. These ways will go a long way in helping to restore our capacity in physical and emotional health.

Conclusion

A lot of people, as have been mentioned above, have lots of problems that are associated with dysfunction of the tenth cranial nerve. However, we often make a mistake when experiencing several symptoms, for instance, epilepsy of attacking the symptoms alone and not the root cause. In most cases, as seen in the case of epilepsy and depression, among other things, the primary reason for these is a malfunction of the vagus nerve.

In addition, usually, going through the conventional means of alleviating the symptoms of certain diseases and ailments only have temporary effects as patients have to manage the symptoms of these diseases throughout their lives. However, this book offers practical and straightforward ways by which the symptoms of these diseases can be alleviated. These methods are practical exercises that have specific instructions that are to be carried out meticulously to get the best results

When you begin these exercises, it is recommended that you record the progress you are making and take down any signs or issues that disturb you. It is also recommended to look at the symbols listed in the first part of this book. Afterward, note how frequently a symptom has occurred and indicate how strong it is. Afterward, you can then look back and observe the changes.

As a therapist, too, you also have to be skilled in carrying out these exercises and monitoring the progress of your patients. By being skilled in carrying out these exercises, you would be able to carry out these exercises better and restore normal vagal function in your patients.

Conclusively, it is essential to note that as effective as these exercises are, it is crucial to pick the one that suits you and the condition that you wish to correct best. By this, you will get the best out of the exercises and access the healing power of the tenth cranial nerve. Remember, reading about the drills that restore normal vagal function is not enough, practicing the exercises judiciously is what brings about the results.

Made in the USA
Middletown, DE
01 February 2020